The
ECG
in Emergency
Decision
Making

The ECG

in Emergency Decision Making

Hein J. J. Wellens, M.D.
Professor and Chairman
Department of Cardiology
Academic Hospital Maastricht
University of Limburg
Maastricht, The Netherlands

Mary Boudreau Conover, R.N., B.S.N.Ed.
Director of Education
Critical Care Conferences
Santa Cruz, California

W.B. SAUNDERS COMPANY
A Division of Harcourt Brace & Company
Philadelphia ■ London ■ Toronto ■ Montreal ■ Sydney ■ Tokyo

W.B. SAUNDERS COMPANY
A Division of
Harcourt Brace & Company

The Curtis Center
Independence Square West
Philadelphia, Pennsylvania 19106-3399

Library of Congress Cataloging-in-Publication Data

Wellens, H. J. J.

The ECG in emergency decision making/Hein J. J. Wellens,
Mary Boudreau Conover.
    p. cm.
Includes bibliographical references.
IBN 0–7216–3214–9

1. Electrocardiography   2. Heart—Diseases.   3. Medical
   emergencies.   I. Conover, Mary Boudreau.
   II. Title. [DNLM: 1. Electrocardiography. 2. Emergencies.
   3. Heart Diseases—diagnosis. WG 140 W447e]

RC683.5.E5W39   1992

616.1′207′547—dc20

DNLM/DLC   91–21432

Editor: Michael Brown
Designer: Bill Donnelly
Production Manager: Peter Faber
Manuscript Editor: Karen Okie
Illustration Coordinator: Lisa Lambert
Indexer: Susan Thomas
Cover Designer: Michelle Maloney

The ECG in Emergency Decision Making   ISBN 0–7216–3214–9

Printed in the United States of America.

Last digit is the print number: 9   8   7   6   5   4   3

Preface

In cardiac emergencies, the correct diagnosis of the underlying cause is the first step to optimal treatment. This book discusses the importance of an informed and systematic approach to the 12-lead electrocardiogram (ECG) for accurate and effective decision-making in cardiac emergencies. Correct treatment based on an understanding of the mechanism that caused the cardiac emergency may not only be lifesaving in the immediate situation but may also improve the quality of life.

Presented here in an easily understood format are concise and logical steps to the ECG recognition of the underlying mechanism of cardiac emergencies, their prognostic significance, and the best treatment. The reader should be comfortable with the basics of electrocardiography for maximal benefit.

Each chapter begins with a brief, highlighted summary section that clearly outlines a systematic, step-by-step approach to correct diagnosis and treatment. In the remainder of the chapter these steps are fully developed, leading to correct interpretation and understanding of the ECG changes observed in certain emergency situations.

At the present time, aggressive therapy in acute myocardial infarction, including administration of thrombolytic agents, early coronary angiography, balloon angioplasty, and coronary bypass surgery, is determined by the amount of heart muscle threatened by the myocardial infarction. The ECG guidelines that identify patients who will profit most from thrombolytic therapy are given in Chapter 1. This chapter also covers the importance of lead V_{4R} and the necessity of recognizing the development of bundle branch block as means of identifying high-risk patients.

Chapter 2 discusses the ECG from patients with chest pain of recent onset. You will learn how to recognize severe main-stem or three-vessel disease and a critical narrowing high in the left anterior descending coronary artery.

New clues to QRS morphology described in Chapter 3 provide accurate and rapid recognition of ventricular tachycardia, while Chapter 4 gives a systematic approach to the differentiation among the mechanisms of paroxysmal supraventricular tachycardia. The remaining chapters contain step-by-step emergency approaches to slow atrial rhythms, atrioventricular block, acute pulmonary embolism, drug-related emergencies, potassium derangements, and the emergencies that are encountered in patients with pace-makers and in the prehospital setting.

The appendices contribute a valuable reference for necessary emergency skills, such as rapid determination of the QRS axis, correct procedures for defibrillation and emergency cardioversion, and dosing of emergency cardiac drugs.

Appendix 4 provides a table for quick reference to the minimal number of leads required for a diagnosis in a given clinical setting. It is highly recommended and advantageous to record 12-lead ECGs in all patients with rhythm disturbances. However, because of equipment limitations in many critical care units and emergency rooms, we are aware that this is not always possible. We have therefore included comments in the text and a table in the Appendix to guide you in your selection of leads.

How to perform carotid sinus massage, information about other vagal maneuvers, and the proper physical examination of patients during tachy-cardia are described in the two chapters on tachycardias.

Prehospital emergencies are covered, with an emphasis on the impor-tance of a systematic, accurate, and early enroute and emergency department response to acute myocardial infarction, unstable angina, tachycardia, and bradycardia.

We strongly believe that correct interpretation of the ECG in the emergency situation leads to a better outcome for many of our patients. We therefore hope that the information presented in this book will challenge, motivate, and help those caring for the patient under these emergency cardiac conditions.

HEIN J.J. WELLENS, M.D.
MARY B. CONOVER, R.N., B.S.N.Ed.

Acknowledgments

Many colleagues from the Maastricht group contributed ECGs for this book. They are, in alphabetical order, Frits Bär, Simon Braat, Pedro Brugada, Emiel Cheriex, Karel den Dulk, Herman Frank, Anton Gorgels, Johan Janssen, Vincent van Ommen, Frans Pieters, Jacques Schmitz, Joep Smeets, Jan Stappers, Hans de Swart, Frank Vermeer, and Chris de Zwaan.

Most of the art work was expertly made by Adri van den Dool. In the preparation of the manuscript, an essential secretarial role was played by Birgit van der Burg and Lenny Frissen. The help and continuous support of all these people are gratefully acknowledged!

HEIN J. J. WELLENS, M.D.
MARY B. CONOVER, R.N., B.S.N.Ed.

Contents

CHAPTER

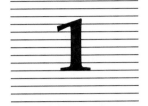

1

Acute Myocardial Infarction

EMERGENCY DECISIONS

1. Ascertain the time from onset of pain.
2. Evaluate 12-lead ECG for:
   Type of myocardial infarction (anterior or inferior)
   ST segment elevation score
   Q waves
   Bundle branch block and hemiblock to identify patients at high risk of dying early; such patients should be managed aggressively.
3. Identify candidates for thrombolytic therapy (ST segment elevation score; how much and in how many leads?).
4. In inferior wall myocardial infarction, record lead V_4R.

IDENTIFICATION OF CANDIDATES FOR THROMBOLYTIC THERAPY

In the patient admitted because of acute myocardial infarction, recognition of the area at risk is of utmost importance; its size and location determine aggressiveness of therapy and help in selecting patients most likely to profit from thrombolytic therapy.[1]

It is important to rule out patients who will not benefit from thrombolytic therapy, because such patients should not be subjected to the risk of bleeding and the need for blood transfusions associated with thrombolysis. In this section we offer a systematic approach by which those patients with acute myocardial infarction who are most likely to benefit from thrombolytic therapy before or at the time of admission can be quickly identified.

Thrombolytic therapy is most beneficial in patients with acute myocardial infarction admitted soon after the onset of chest pain with signs of a large infarction (development of Q waves) or extensive ischemic areas (high ST segment elevation or marked ST depression in several ECG leads).[2, 3]

1

TIME FROM ONSET OF PAIN

Significant infarction size limitation occurs in patients arriving at the hospital within 2 hours after the onset of chest pain.[4-6] If thrombolysis is initiated within 1 hour after the onset of chest pain, infarction size is reduced by 50 percent and if initiated between 1 and 2 hours, infarction size is reduced by 30 percent. If patients are admitted between 2 and 4 hours after the onset of pain, infarction size is reduced by only 13 percent; in fact, in a subgroup of these patients there was no limitation of infarction size in spite of the fact that successful reperfusion was achieved.[2]

After a delay of more than 4 hours from onset of pain, the value of thrombolytic therapy is less clear. It still seems useful in anterior infarction with a high ST score and Q waves. Recent studies suggest that even at a later stage patients may still benefit from thrombolytic therapy because of a lower incidence of left ventricular dilatation and ventricular arrhythmias.[7-9]

It should be noted that acute pericarditis can be the cause of the subjective symptoms of acute myocardial infarction as well as an ECG pattern with a high ST segment score.

ST SEGMENT SCORING

In both anterior and inferior acute myocardial infarction the greatest reduction of infarction size by thrombolytic therapy is achieved in patients with the largest infarctions. The amount of ST segment elevation and depression and the number of leads in which these changes are present are proportionate to infarction size; the higher the ST segment elevation, the deeper the ST depression, and the more leads showing these changes, the larger the infarction.[2, 3] Patients most likely to profit from thrombolytic therapy can therefore be recognized by using an ST segment scoring system.[2, 3]

Anterior Wall Myocardial Infarction. For ST segment scoring in anterior wall infarction, add the total amount (in millimeters) of ST elevation in the precordial leads (V_1–V_6). A total of 12 mm or more is a high ST segment score and indicates extensive anterior wall infarction; a low ST segment score in the precordial leads is less than 12 mm.[2]

Inferior Wall Myocardial Infarction. For ST segment scoring in inferior wall infarction, add the total amount (in millimeters) of ST segment elevation in the inferior leads (II, III, and aVF). A total of 7 mm or more is a high ST segment score and indicates extensive inferior wall infarction; a low ST segment score in the inferior leads is less than 7 mm.

SIGNIFICANCE OF Q WAVES

Although in the past Q waves have been thought to indicate myocardial necrosis, it is now known that extensive ischemia can result in transient Q waves due to conduction delay in the zone under that electrode.[10] It has been shown that significant myocardial salvage by thrombolysis can be accomplished in patients with new pathological Q waves; even after 2 hours the infarction size can be limited by therapy, indicating that large anterior wall infarctions are still evolving at that time. Thus, patients should not be excluded from thrombolytic therapy simply because Q waves are present. When there is little ST segment elevation in anterior wall myocardial infarction (less than 12 mm total in precordial leads), and the absence of Q waves indicates that thrombolysis is not required, spontaneous reperfusion may have already taken place.

INFORMATION NEEDED

1. Time from onset of pain (0–2 hr; 2–4 hr; >4 hr)
2. Infarction location (anterior or inferoposterior)
3. ST segment elevation score
4. Presence or absence of Q waves
5. Lead V_4R in inferior wall infarction

Table 1–1 simplifies the identification of candidates most likely to profit from thrombolytic therapy. If the ST segment score is *high* and the delay less than 2 hours, all patients with myocardial infarction are candidates; if the delay is 2 to 4 hours, the best candidates for thrombolysis are:

1. All patients who have myocardial infarction and do not have Q waves
2. All patients with anterior wall infarction with Q waves

If the ST score is *low*, only patients with anterior wall infarction and Q waves will have reduction of infarction size from thrombolysis up to 4 hours after the onset of pain.

Figure 1–1 is a 12-lead ECG from a patient with acute inferior wall infarction and was recorded less than 2 hours after the onset of pain. It illustrates a case where use of thrombolytics will result in marked reduction in infarction size. After 2 hours the patients with inferior wall myocardial infarction most likely to profit from thrombolysis are those with high ST segment scores and no Q waves.[2]

Figure 1–2 is the 12-lead ECG from a patient with acute anteroseptal myocardial infarction recorded less than 2 hours after the onset of pain. The high ST segment score (more than 25 mm) is a clear indication for thrombolytic therapy. Had this patient been seen more than 2 hours from the onset of pain, thrombolysis would still have been indicated.

Table 1–1. **Candidates Most Likely to Profit from Thrombolytic Therapy**

Delay	High ST Segment Elevation Score*	Low ST Segment Elevation Score†
<2 hr	All patients with MI‡	Anterior MI with Q waves
2–4 hr	Anterior MI‡ (with and without Q waves) Inferior MI without Q waves	Anterior MI with Q waves

*>12 mm, leads V_1–V_6; ≥7 mm, leads II, III, aVF.
†<12 mm, leads V_1–V_6; <7 mm, leads II, III, aVF.
‡MI = myocardial infarction.

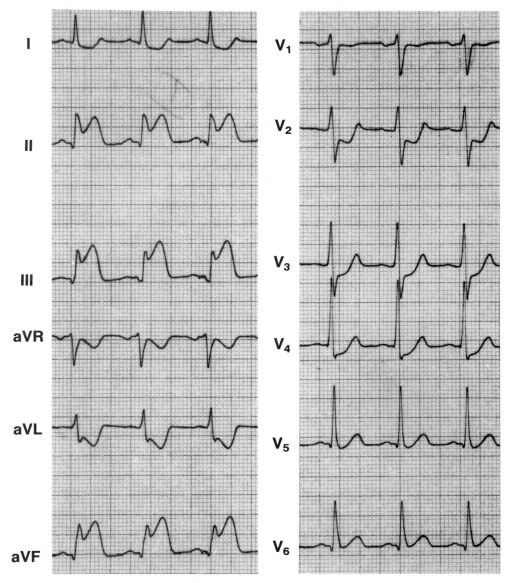

Figure 1–1. Acute inferior wall myocardial infarction with a high ST score less than 2 hours after the onset of pain. The ST score in leads II, III, and aVF is 13 mm; small Q waves are present. This patient is a candidate for thrombolysis. The additional recording of lead V₄R should have been of help to identify the coronary artery involved, presence of right ventricular infarction, and risk of developing AV nodal block.

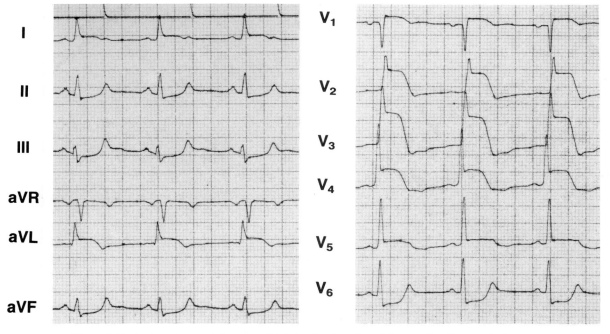

Figure 1–2. Acute anteroseptal myocardial infarction less than 2 hours after the onset of pain. The ST segment score is high and thrombolytic therapy is indicated.

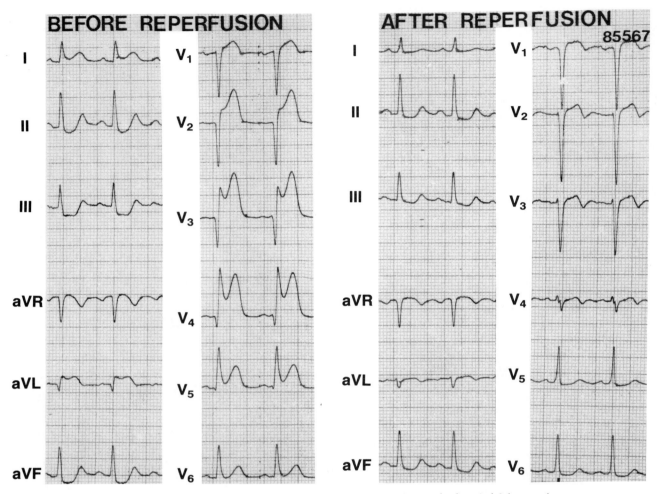

Figure 1–3. Acute anteroseptal infarction in a patient presenting to the hospital 2 hours after the onset of chest pain. Note the presence of Q waves in leads V_2 to V_4 *(left panel)*. Following successful thrombolytic therapy these Q waves disappear *(right panel)*, indicating that the tissue was still salvageable.

Figure 1–3 is an example of how Q waves, which are present during acute ischemia, may disappear after successful reperfusion; the figure underscores the fact that Q waves present in the acute stage of myocardial infarction do not necessarily indicate necrotic and unsalvageable myocardial muscle.

VALUE OF LEAD V_4R IN ACUTE INFERIOR MYOCARDIAL INFARCTION

Lead V_4R identifies:

1. The coronary artery occluded
2. Presence or absence of right ventricular infarction

3. Those at risk for atrioventricular (AV) block
4. Those who will profit most from thrombolytic therapy

Occlusion Sites. With lead V_4R it is possible to identify the occlusion sites in the setting of acute inferior wall myocardial infarction. Figure 1–4 illustrates that in lead V_4R the ST segment is elevated in proximal right coronary artery occlusion; it is not elevated but coves into a positive T wave in distal right coronary artery occlusion; and for a circumflex artery occlusion the T wave is inverted.[11]

High-Risk Patients. The value of thrombolytic therapy in acute myocardial infarction relates to the area at risk and the delay before instituting such therapy. When thrombolytic therapy is being considered for patients with acute inferior wall myocardial infarction, ECG identification of right ventricular infarction identifies the patient who might require more aggressive therapy when intravenous thrombolytic therapy is not successful. More aggressive therapy includes percutaneous transluminal coronary angioplasty (PTCA).

Approximately 45 percent of patients with acute inferoposterior myocardial infarction have right ventricular involvement, and only 5 to 10 percent of these have the hemodynamic picture of right ventricular infarction (low cardiac output and elevated right-sided pressures).[12, 13]

Right Ventricular Infarction. ST segment elevation of 1 mm or more in lead V_4R has a high sensitivity and specificity for detecting right ventricular

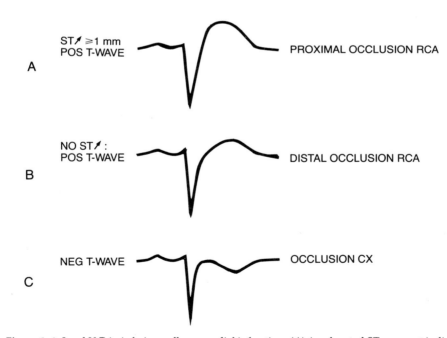

Figure 1–4. Lead V_4R in inferior wall myocardial infarction. *(A)* An elevated ST segment indicates proximal right coronary artery occlusion and right ventricular infarction, and it identifies patients at risk for AV nodal block. *(B)* An ST segment that coves into a positive T wave, without ST segment elevation, identifies distal right coronary artery occlusion (RCA). *(C)* An ST segment that slopes into a negative T wave points to circumflex artery (CX) occlusion.

infarction,[10, 11] pinpointing the site of occlusion in the proximal right coronary artery,[10, 11] and identifying patients at high risk (45%) of developing AV block. In all patients with inferior wall myocardial infarction the incidence of AV block is 15 percent.[13, 14]

Figure 1–5 illustrates the ECG in acute inferoposterior and right ventricular infarction. The ST segment elevation in the inferior leads (II, III, and aVF) indicates inferior wall involvement; the ST segment depression in leads V_1 to V_5 indicates acute posterior wall infarction; and the elevated ST segment

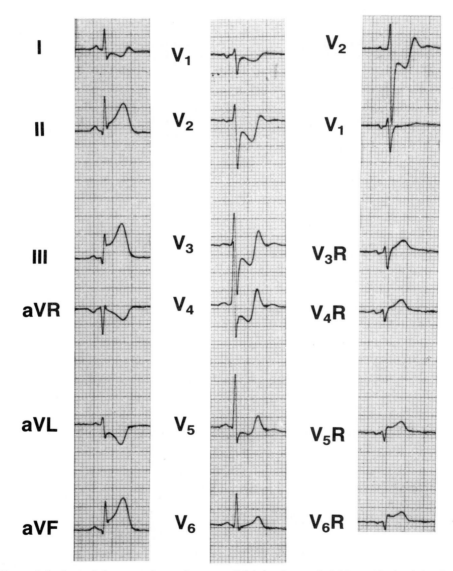

Figure 1–5. Acute inferoposterior wall myocardial infarction and right ventricular infarction. Note the elevated ST segment in lead V_4R, indicating an occlusion in the proximal right coronary artery and right ventricular involvement.

in V_4R indicates right ventricular infarction and proximal right coronary artery occlusion.

An Early Sign. The ST segment elevation in lead V_4R usually disappears within 10 hours after the onset of pain, and thus it is important to record this lead on admission. Figure 1–6 demonstrates the loss of the telltale ST segment elevation in lead V_4R within the span of 6 hours. A recording of lead V_4R at 11 a.m. shows ST segment elevation consistent with right ventricular infarction and proximal right coronary occlusion. This sign has completely disappeared 6 hours later.[13]

Onset chest pain 9:30am

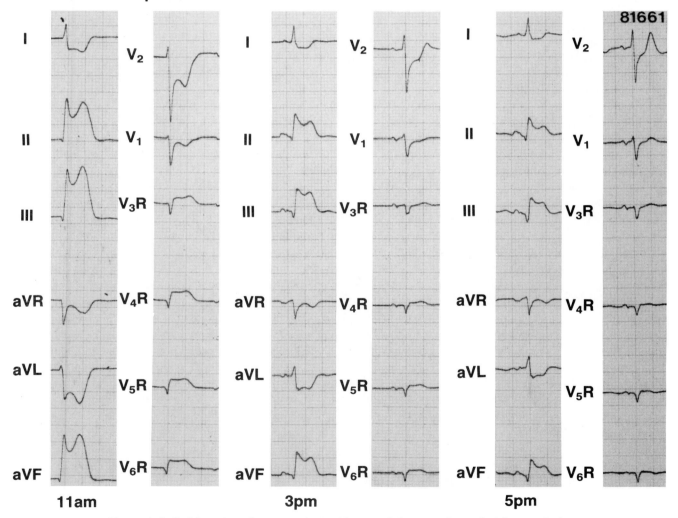

Figure 1–6. Serial tracings from a patient with acute inferoposterior and right ventricular infarction. Note that the diagnostic changes for right ventricular infarction seen in lead V_4R have disappeared 7½ hours after the onset of pain.

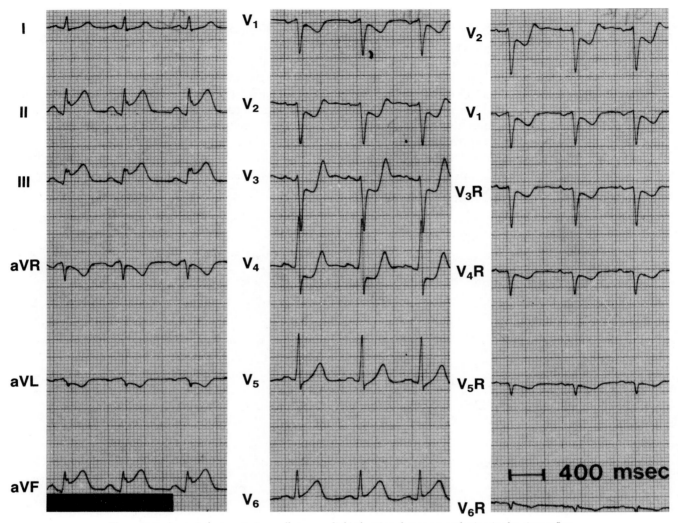

Figure 1–7. Acute inferoposterior wall myocardial infarction due to an occlusion in the circumflex artery. Note in lead V_4R the downsloping of the ST segment into a negative T wave.

Figure 1–7 shows acute inferoposterior wall infarction in a patient with a downsloping ST segment in lead V_4R, indicating a circumflex artery occlusion.

ECG SIGNS OF REPERFUSION

Apart from a decrease in ST segment elevation, the accelerated idioventricular rhythm has been shown to be a sign of reperfusion (spontaneous or as a result of thrombolytic therapy) during acute myocardial infarction.[15] Approx-

imately one-half of the patients with reperfusion have an accelerated idioventricular rhythm when the ECG is recorded continuously following thrombolytic therapy. This finding is of practical clinical importance in that it may
help to identify both spontaneous and thrombolytic-induced reperfusion in
the absence of coronary angiography. As shown by Gorgels,[16] an accelerated
idioventricular rhythm after myocardial infarction indicates not only reperfusion, but also myocardial necrosis.

CHARACTERISTICS OF THE REPERFUSION ARRHYTHMIA

1. Three or more successive ventricular ectopic beats
2. Rate: 50 to 120 beats per minute
3. Onset: After a long coupling interval

An accelerated idioventricular rhythm, as shown in Figure 1–8A, begins
with a long coupling interval. The first few beats are often fusion beats
because the ectopic rhythm emerges when its rate is about the same as that
of the sinus rhythm. This type of ventricular rhythm should be distinguished
from the one beginning with a short coupling interval that is sometimes
called "slow ventricular tachycardia"[17] (Fig. 1–8B), which is frequently
irregular and occurs during the first 24 hours of infarction, but after the
reperfusion phase.

IDENTIFICATION OF THE AREA OF REPERFUSION

The QRS configuration of the accelerated idioventricular rhythm may be of
help in noninvasive identification of the area supplied by the previously
occluded vessel using the following clues:

1. Multiple QRS configurations during the accelerated idioventricular
rhythm frequently accompany reperfusion of the left anterior descending
(LAD) coronary artery; the QRS may be relatively narrow.
2. A V_1-negative configuration excludes a circumflex lesion.
3. An electrical axis between 0 and 180 degrees virtually rules out the
right coronary artery as the infarct artery.[14, 15]

CONDUCTION BLOCKS IN ACUTE
MYOCARDIAL INFARCTION (See also Chapter 6)

The emergence of conduction disturbances between atrium and ventricle in
the acute phase of myocardial infarction is of great prognostic and therapeutic
significance and should therefore be recognized immediately.

The site of block in the AV conduction system (AV node or bundle
branches) is related to which coronary artery is occluded during myocardial
infarction.

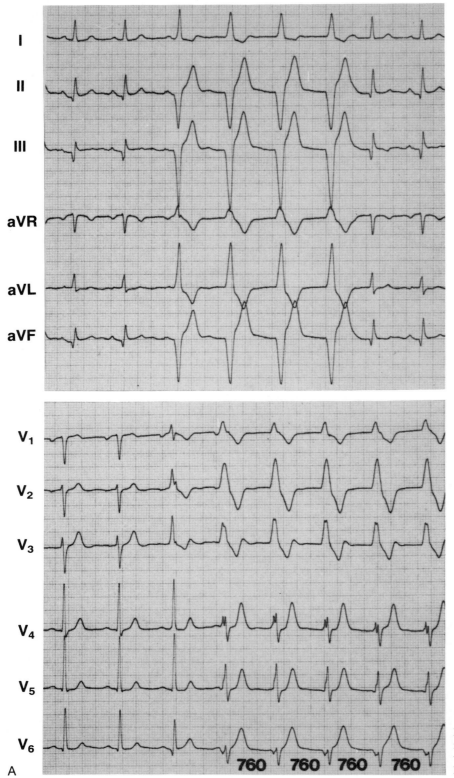

Figure 1–8. *(A)* Accelerated idioventricular rhythm—a reperfusion arrhythmia in a patient with acute inferior wall infarction. Note the long coupling interval.

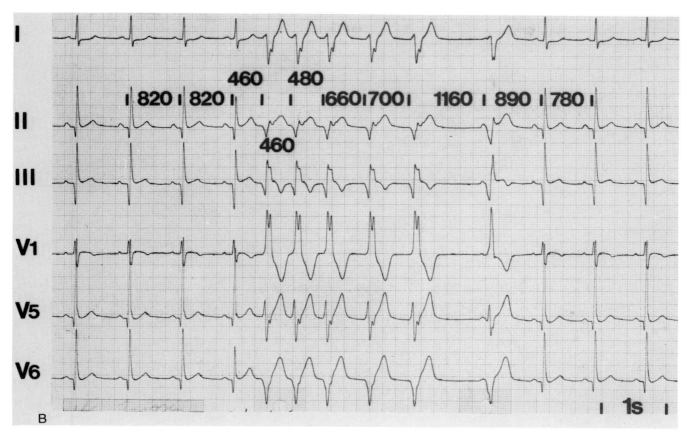

Figure 1–8 *Continued (B)* Example of a slow ventricular tachycardia. Note the shorter coupling interval and the irregular rhythm.

ANATOMY OF THE AV CONDUCTION SYSTEM

As shown in Figure 1–9, the AV conduction system consists of the AV node, the bundle of His, and the specialized intraventricular conduction system. The latter consists mainly of three fascicles—the right bundle branch and the left bundle branch with its two main divisions (anterior and posterior fascicles). The posterior fascicle is usually broad and short, and the right bundle branch and the left anterior fascicle are long and thin.

BLOOD SUPPLY TO THE CONDUCTION SYSTEM

As illustrated in Figure 1–9, in 90 percent of people the right coronary artery, by way of its posterior descending branch, perfuses the posterior one-third of the interventricular conduction system. The AV nodal branch is the main blood supply to the AV node and proximal part of the bundle of His. In some people the AV nodal artery also supplies the distal portion of the His bundle and the proximal bundle branches.[18, 19]

The LAD coronary artery and its branches supply the anterior wall of

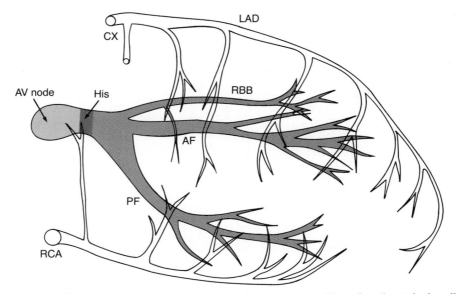

Figure 1–9. The trifascicular intraventricular conduction system. Note that the right bundle branch (RBB) and the superior division of the left bundle branch (AF) are both anterior structures and therefore are vulnerable in anteroseptal myocardial infarction. The posterior division of the left bundle branch (PF) is broad and supplied by both the left anterior descending (LAD) and the right coronary artery (RCA).

the heart and the anterior two-thirds of the septum. In most hearts, the first septal perforator of the LAD is the main blood supply to the distal part of the bundle of His and the proximal bundle branches.[18]

AV NODAL BLOCK

Clinical Implications. The right coronary artery usually supplies the AV node, and obstruction of that artery causes inferior myocardial infarction, frequently leading to AV nodal conduction disturbances. In acute inferior wall infarction, ST segment elevation in lead V_4R identifies patients having proximal obstruction in the right coronary artery and an almost 50 percent chance of developing high-degree (second-degree or more) AV nodal block (Fig. 1–10).

Prognosis. When high-degree AV nodal block occurs in acute inferior myocardial infarction (which is the case in 15 percent of patients) the inhospital mortality rate is two and one-half times that of inferior wall infarction without high-degree AV block.[20] This increased mortality is probably the result of the proximal location of the obstruction in the right coronary artery leading to a large inferior wall infarction with right ventricular involvement. These AV nodal conduction disturbances are transient, usually disappearing after a few days; in exceptional cases they may last for a few weeks. The escape pacemaker during complete AV nodal block is located

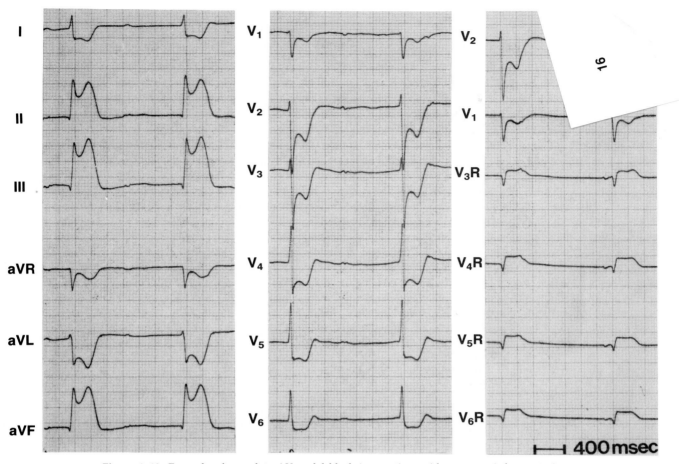

Figure 1–10. Example of complete AV nodal block in a patient with an acute inferoposterior myocardial infarction and right ventricular involvement.

just below the AV node,[21] and it usually produces an acceptable and dependable rhythm at a rate of 40 to 60 beats per minute.

Treatment. Atropine or temporary transvenous pacing is indicated in case of (1) Adams-Stokes attacks, (2) a low ventricular rate accompanied by congestive failure, and/or (3) bradycardia-dependent ventricular arrhythmias.

BUNDLE BRANCH BLOCK AND HEMIBLOCK

Clinical Implications. The development of bundle branch block and hemiblock during the acute phase of myocardial infarction indicates extensive anterior wall infarction, because such conduction problems indicate an occlusion proximally in the LAD coronary artery. Before the introduction of thrombolytic therapy this complication occurred in 10 percent of patients with an acute anterior wall myocardial infarction. The inhospital mortality was around 55 percent, which is four times higher than that in patients not developing bundle branch block.[22] Although exact figures are not yet available, the clinical impression is that following the introduction of thrombolytic therapy, the incidence of bundle branch block after acute anterior wall myocardial infarction decreased.

Prognosis. When anterior wall myocardial infarction is complicated by bundle branch block and hemiblock, early death occurs because of pump failure and ventricular tachycardia or fibrillation. Death from pump failure occurs within a few days. If the patient survives the critical early days, there is a 30 percent chance that sustained ventricular tachycardia or fibrillation will develop 1 to 2 weeks later.[19, 22, 23] Lie and associates[23] have shown that in this clinical setting (anterior wall myocardial infarction complicated by bundle branch block and hemiblock) there is a high chance of developing complete AV block, which, if the patient survives, is usually transient and requires only a temporary pacemaker.

Treatment. The finding of bundle branch block as a complication of anterior wall infarction calls for aggressive treatment. Intravenous thrombolytic therapy is given; when it is not successful, the patient is taken to the cardiac catheterization laboratory to receive intracoronary thrombolytic therapy. If this treatment fails to open the LAD coronary artery, the thrombus is perforated and emergency PTCA performed. During the same catheterization, a Swan-Ganz catheter and a temporary pacing lead are inserted. The Swan-Ganz catheter will provide information about pump function.

If the patient survives the first few days, continuous rhythm monitoring is still required because of the chance of developing sustained ventricular tachycardia or fibrillation 1 to 2 weeks after the onset of anterior wall myocardial infarction. Table 1–2 summarizes some of the features of AV conduction disturbances complicating myocardial infarction.

Table 1–2. **Features of AV Conduction Disturbances Complicating Acute Myocardial Infarction**

Feature	Inferior MI	Anterior MI
Site of block	AV node	Bundle branches
Artery involved	RCA	LAD
Escape rhythm	Narrow QRS Rate 40–60/minute Dependable	Wide QRS Rate <40/minute Undependable
Duration of block	Transient	Transient
Increase in hospital mortality (compared to same infarction location without block)	2½ times	4 times

Abbreviations: RCA—right coronary artery; LAD—left anterior descending coronary artery; MI—myocardial infarction.

RIGHT BUNDLE BRANCH BLOCK

In acute myocardial infarction the appearance of right bundle branch block is usually associated with distal conduction system block secondary to anterior rather than inferior wall infarction. The risk of progression to complete heart block is twice that of left bundle branch block especially when associated with fascicular block.[19]

ECG RECOGNITION

In right bundle branch block, the QRS pattern in lead V_1 is broad with a terminal R wave (classically the pattern is a triphasic rSR'); in leads I, aVL, and V_6 there is a terminal S wave (qRS). In right bundle branch block secondary to acute anterior wall myocardial infarction, the ventricular complex in lead V_1 looks different than it would had there not been such a complication. That is, because of septal involvement, the initial R wave is missing and the triphasic pattern (rSR') changes to a biphasic pattern (QR). The little q wave in lead V_6 that reflects normal septal activation is also absent.

In Figure 1–11, the pattern on the left shows the classic pattern of right bundle branch block (rSR' pattern in lead V_1 and a qRS pattern in lead V_6) in a patient with inferior myocardial infarction. In this case, the right bundle branch block was present before myocardial infarction occurred. The pattern on the right is an example of anteroseptal myocardial infarction complicated by right bundle branch block. Note the loss of the initial r wave in precordial leads V_1 to V_5; this reflects a loss of anterior forces.

MECHANISM

In right bundle branch block the two ventricles are activated one after the other instead of simultaneously. Septal and left ventricular activation proceed normally; the sole abnormality is late activation of the right ventricle, which explains the late R in lead V_1 and the S wave in leads I, aVL, and V_6 (Fig. 1–12). However, in acute anteroseptal infarction the septal forces are lost and lead V_1 shows a QR pattern (Fig. 1–12).

LEFT BUNDLE BRANCH BLOCK

In acute myocardial infarction, left bundle branch block (LBBB) may occur secondary to inferior and anterior wall myocardial infarction because the main stem of the left bundle branch may receive blood supply from either the AV nodal or the LAD coronary arteries. When ischemic heart disease is excluded, left bundle branch block is usually associated with hypertensive, primary, or degenerative myocardial disease.[19, 23, 24]

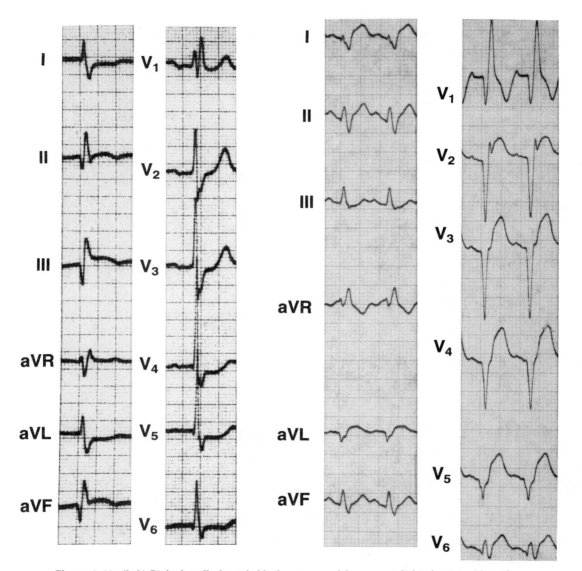

Figure 1–11. *(Left)* Right bundle branch block not caused by myocardial infarction. Note the classic rSR′ pattern in lead V_1 and the qRS pattern in lead V_6. The patient has an inferior wall infarction. *(Right)* Right bundle branch block caused by anteroseptal myocardial infarction. Note qR pattern in lead V_1.

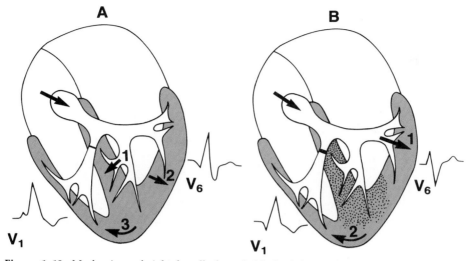

Figure 1–12. Mechanism of right bundle branch block. *(A)* Note that the right ventricle is activated last and without any opposing forces, resulting in the late R' in lead V_1 and the S wave in lead V_6. In anteroseptal infarction *(B)* a QR pattern develops in lead V_1. Loss of anterior wall tissue causes an R/S pattern in lead V_6.

ECG RECOGNITION

In left bundle branch block, the QRS complex in lead V_1 is broad and negative (QS or rS). In leads I, aVL, and V_6 the complex is totally positive (no q and no s). These features are seen in Figure 1–13. The intrinsicoid deflection over the left ventricle (V_6) is delayed. If the left bundle branch block is associated with anteroseptal infarction, a Q wave may be present in leads I, aVL, V_5, and V_6 (Fig. 1–14).

MECHANISM

The sequence of ventricular activation during left bundle branch block is totally different from that during normal conduction. The normal narrow QRS reflects synchronous activation of the ventricles by simultaneous conduction over the right and left bundle branches. When the left bundle is blocked, the impulse reaches the right ventricle first by way of the right bundle branch. Then the septum is activated from right to left, followed by the remainder of the left ventricle. Figure 1–15 compares ventricular activation in left bundle branch block with and without myocardial infarction. Without infarction the septum and right ventricle are activated together; in anteroseptal infarction the right ventricle is activated without opposing septal forces, causing a tall narrow R wave in lead V_1 and a Q wave in lead V_6.

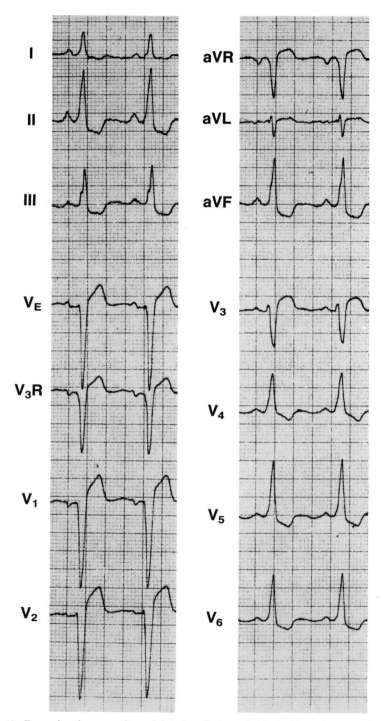

Figure 1–13. Example of uncomplicated left bundle branch block. Note the entirely positive complex in leads I, aVL, and V$_6$, and the negative complex in lead V$_1$.

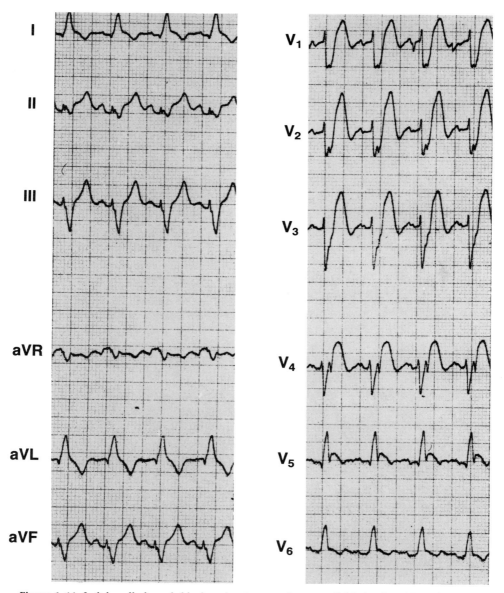

Figure 1–14. Left bundle branch block and anteroseptal myocardial infarction. Note that small Q waves are present in leads I, aVL, V$_5$, and V$_6$.

In lead V$_1$ during left bundle branch block without infarction, an initial small, narrow R wave may be present, probably due to activation of the anterior papillary branch of the right bundle. Because the two ventricles are activated one after the other, first the right ventricle and then the left, the main current goes leftward, away from lead V$_1$. This accounts for the broad negative deflection in that lead and the broad positive one in lead V$_6$.

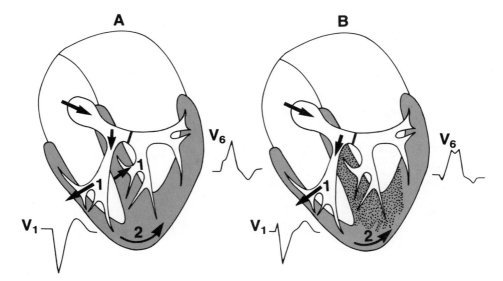

Figure 1–15. Mechanism of left bundle branch block. *(A)* Ventricular activation goes from right to left to produce a negative QRS complex in lead V_1 and a positive complex in lead V_6. In anteroseptal infarction *(B)* early unopposed right ventricular activation produces the initial R in lead V_1 and a Q in lead V_6.

If left bundle branch block develops secondary to a large anteroseptal infarction, loss of septal tissue and late left ventricular activation cause unopposed right ventricular activation, causing the QRS to have an initial narrow R wave in lead V_1 and a Q wave in lead V_6 (Fig. 1–15).

LEFT ANTERIOR HEMIBLOCK

Left anterior hemiblock may occur secondary to anterior wall myocardial infarction.

ECG RECOGNITION

In left anterior hemiblock there is left axis deviation of -30 degrees and a small q wave in leads I and aVL (Fig. 1–16). The QRS duration is not prolonged beyond normal.[25]

MECHANISM

The anterior fascicle of the conduction system is relatively thin and therefore vulnerable to injury. A block in this division of the left bundle branch results in delayed activation (40 msec) of the anterolateral area of the left ventricle,

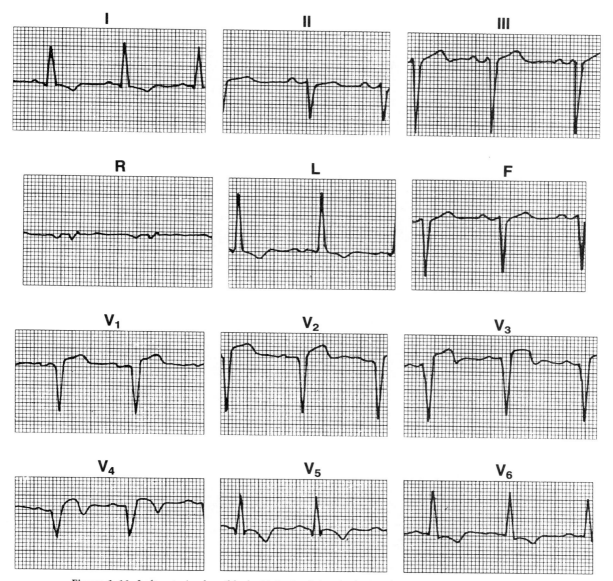

Figure 1–16. Left anterior hemiblock. Note the left axis deviation, the small q in leads I and aVL, and the small r wave in lead II.

causing marked left axis deviation because the impulse activates the left ventricle through the posterior fascicle, spreading upward and to the left.[10]

LEFT POSTERIOR HEMIBLOCK

Left posterior hemiblock rarely occurs in the setting of acute myocardial infarction. If it develops associated with right bundle branch block, it

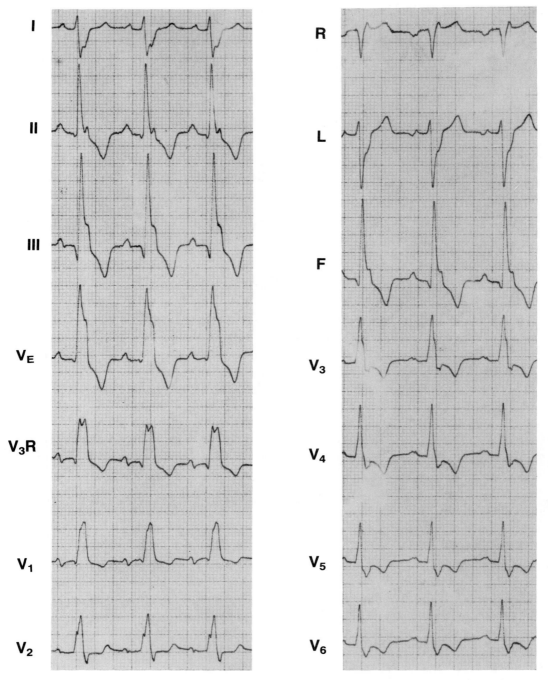

Figure 1–17. Left posterior hemiblock. Note the right axis deviation, the small r in leads I and aVL, and the small q in lead II. In this patient complete right bundle branch block is also present.

indicates a poor prognosis because, as shown in Figure 1–9, this requires occlusion in both the LAD and the right coronary arteries.

ECG RECOGNITION

With left posterior hemiblock there is right axis deviation of greater than +120 degrees and a small r wave in leads I and aVL (Fig. 1–17).

MECHANISM

A block in the posterior fascicle causes marked right axis deviation because the impulse activates the left ventricle through only the anterior fascicle, spreading downward and to the right and causing lead I to be mainly negative and leads II, III, and aVF to be mainly positive. The initial forces (first 0.02 sec) travel from the anterior papillary muscle, upward and leftward. This is why there is a small initial r wave in leads I and aVL and a q wave in leads II, III, and aVF.

SUMMARY

The treatment of acute myocardial infarction has changed dramatically with the introduction of thrombolytic therapy and the availability of other methods of reperfusion, such as PTCA and emergency coronary artery bypass surgery.

Essential in the management of acute myocardial infarction is stratification according to infarction location and size and time interval between onset of pain to admission.

The 12-lead ECG is of great value in (1) making decisions as to the necessity of thrombolytic therapy (using ST-T segment score and presence or absence of Q waves); (2) recognizing reperfusion (by the appearance of accelerated idioventricular rhythm); (3) diagnosing the site of occlusion in the coronary artery responsible for inferoposterior infarction; (4) identifying right ventricular involvement; (5) recognizing patients with inferoposterior infarction at high risk for developing AV nodal block; and (6) risk stratification because of the emergence of AV conduction disturbances.

The bundle branches receive their blood supply from the same artery that supplies the anterior wall of the heart. Thus, bundle branch block and hemiblock are serious complications of acute anterior wall myocardial infarction. Prognosis in these patients is mainly determined by their extensive anterior wall infarction, which may lead to pump failure and early death due to ventricular tachycardia and fibrillation. There is a high incidence of complete AV block in patients with anterior wall infarction who develop right bundle branch block and hemiblock. Complete block, however, is usually transient, and if the patient survives the acute phase and the ventricular tachycardia and ventricular fibrillation that often develop 1 to 2 weeks later, implantation of a permanent pacemaker is rarely needed.

References

1. Verheugt, F.W.A., van Eenige, M.J., Res, J., et al.: Bleeding complications of intracoronary fibrinolytic therapy in acute myocardial infarction. Br. Heart J. 54:455, 1985.
2. Bar, F.W., Vermeer, F., de Zwaan, C., et al.: Value of admission electrocardiogram in predicting outcome of thrombolytic therapy in acute myocardial infarction. Am. J. Cardiol. 59:6, 1987.
3. Clemmensen, P., Grande, P., Saunamäki, K., et al.: Effect of intravenous streptokinase on the relation between initial ST predicted size and final QRS estimated size of acute myocardial infarction. J. Am. Coll. Cardiol. 16:1252–1257, 1990.
4. Gruppo Italiano per lo Studio della Streptochinasi nel' Infarto miocardico (GISSI): Long-term effects of intravenous thrombolysis in acute myocardial infarction, final report of the GISSI study. Lancet 2:871–874, 1987.
5. Simoons, M.L., Serruys, P.W., Brand, M.V.D., et al.: Early thrombolysis in acute myocardial infarction: Limitation of infarct size and improved survival. J. Am. Coll. Cardiol. 7:717–728, 1986.
6. Vermeer, F., Simoons, M.L., Bar, F.W., et al.: Which patients benefit most from early thrombolytic therapy with intracoronary streptokinase? Circulation 74:1379–1389, 1986.
7. ISIS Collaborative Group: Randomized trial of intravenous streptokinase, oral aspirin, both or neither among 17,187 cases of suspected acute myocardial infarction. Lancet 2:349–360, 1988.
8. Braunwald, E.: Myocardial reperfusion, reduction of infarct size, reduction of left ventricular dysfunction, and improved survival: Should the paradigm be expanded? Circulation 79:441–444, 1989.
9. Lavie, C.J., O'Keefe, J.H., Chesebro, J.H., et al.: Prevention of late ventricular dilatation after acute myocardial infarction by successful thrombolytic reperfusion. J. Am. Coll. Cardiol. 16:31–36, 1990.
10. Durrer, D., van Dam, R.T., Freud, G.E., et al.: Total excitation of the isolated human heart. Circulation 41:895, 1970.
11. Braat, S.H., Gorgels, A.P.M., Bar, F.W., et al.: Value of the ST-T segment in lead V_4R in inferior wall acute myocardial infarction to predict the site of coronary arterial occlusion. Am. J. Cardiol. 62:140–142, 1988.
12. Braat, S.H., Brugada, P., de Zwaan, C., et al.: Value of electrocardiogram in diagnosing right ventricular involvement in patients with an acute inferior wall myocardial infarction. Br. Heart J. 49:368–372, 1983.
13. Wellens, H.J.J.: The electrocardiogram 80 years after Einthoven. J. Am. Coll. Cardiol. 7:484–491, 1986.
14. Braat, S.H., de Zwaan, C., Brugada, P., et al.: Right ventricular involvement with acute inferior wall myocardial infarction identifies high risk of developing atrioventricular nodal conduction disturbances. Am. Heart J. 107:1183, 1984.
15. Goldberg, S., Greenspan, A.J., Urban, P.L., et al.: Reperfusion arrhythmia: A marker of restoration of anterograde flow during intracoronary thrombolysis for acute myocardial infarction. Am. Heart J. 105:26–32, 1983.
16. Gorgels, A.P.M., Vos, M.A., Letsch, I.S., et al.: Usefulness of the accelerated idioventricular rhythm as a marker for myocardial necrosis and reperfusion during thrombolytic therapy in acute myocardial infarction. Am. J. Cardiol. 61:231–235, 1988.
17. Sclarovsky, S., Strasberg, B., Fuchs, J., et al.: Multiform accelerated idioventricular rhythm in acute myocardial infarction: Electrocardiographic characteristics and response to verapamil. Am. J. Cardiol. 52:43–47, 1983.
18. Frink, R.J., and James, T.N.: Normal blood supply to the human His bundle and proximal bundle branches. Circulation 47:8, 1973.
19. Ross, D.L.: Approach to the patient with bundle branch block. In Wellens, H.J.J., and Kulbertus, H.E. (eds.): What's New in Electrocardiography. The Hague, 1981, Martinus Nijhoff.
20. Tans, A.C., and Lie, K.I.: AV nodal block in acute myocardial infarction. In Wellens, H.J.J., Lie, K.I., and Janse, M.J. (eds.): The Conduction System of the Heart. Leiden, 1976, Stenfert Kroese.
21. Rosen, K.M., Loeb, M.S., Chuquimia, R., et al.: Site of heart block in acute myocardial infarction. Circulation 42:925, 1970.
22. Lie, K.I., Wellens, H.J., Schuilenburg, R.M., et al.: Factors influencing prognosis of bundle branch block complicating acute antero-septal infarction. The value of His bundle recordings. Circulation 50:935–941, 1974.
23. Lie, K.I., Wellens, H.J., and Schuilenburg, R.M.: Bundle branch block and acute myocardial infarction. In Wellens, H.J.J., Lie, K.I., and Janse, M.J. (eds.): The Conduction System of

the Heart: Structure, Function, and Clinical Implications. The Hague, 1976, Martinus Nijhoff, p. 662.

24. Schneider, J.F., Thomas, H.E., McNamara, P.M., et al.: Clinical-electrocardiographic correlates of newly acquired left bundle branch block: The Framingham study. Am. J. Cardiol. 55:1332, 1985.

25. Das, G.: Left axis deviation: A spectrum of intraventricular conduction block. Circulation 53:917, 1976.

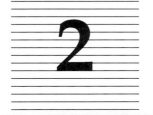

CHAPTER

2

ECG Identification of High-Risk Patients With Unstable Angina

EMERGENCY APPROACH

ECG RECOGNITION OF CRITICAL PROXIMAL LEFT ANTERIOR DESCENDING CORONARY ARTERY STENOSIS IN PATIENTS WITH UNSTABLE ANGINA

- Unstable angina
- No elevation or minimally elevated enzymes
- No pathological precordial Q waves
- ST segment in precordial leads (especially V_2, V_3) isoelectric or slightly elevated (1 mm), concave or straight
- Progressive, symmetrical T wave inversion
- ECG signs appearing during pain-free interval and disappearing during period of chest pain

ECG RECOGNITION OF LEFT MAINSTEM AND THREE-VESSEL DISEASE IN PATIENTS WITH UNSTABLE ANGINA

- Record 12-lead ECG during chest pain because ECG may be normal during pain-free period
- ST segment elevation in leads aVR and V_1
- ST segment depression in eight or more leads

INTRODUCTION

Unstable angina is diagnosed when anginal symptoms that have recently started increase in severity over a short time span. Characteristically, the anginal pain that had occurred at first only during heavy exercise now appears after slight exercise or even at rest. This may happen in patients who have never experienced anginal symptoms and also after a long anginal pain-free interval in patients who have suffered a myocardial infarction in the past.

In patients presenting with unstable angina, it is of the greatest importance to know how large an area of ventricular muscle will be lost when the narrowed coronary artery causing the anginal symptoms becomes occluded. This chapter discusses how the 12-lead ECG can be of great help in identifying patients with unstable angina who are at great risk of losing a considerable amount of myocardium if the process of occlusion is not arrested.

CRITICAL PROXIMAL LEFT ANTERIOR DESCENDING CORONARY ARTERY STENOSIS

Critical stenosis high in the left anterior descending (LAD) coronary artery can be diagnosed in patients with unstable angina from specific ST-T segment changes in precordial leads on or shortly after admission. The presence of such a pattern and corroborative results of subsequent cardiac catheterization signal the need for bypass grafting or percutaneous transvenous coronary angioplasty (PTCA) to prevent the development of extensive anterior wall myocardial infarction. In view of the large area of the ventricle at risk, the recognition of this ECG pattern takes on critical importance.

ECG RECOGNITION

ST-T changes are found in leads V_2 and V_3, as illustrated in Figure 2–1, but they are not necessarily limited to those leads. Notably, there is little or no ST segment elevation (≤ 1 mm), no loss of R wave, and little or no enzyme elevation, but subsequent ECGs show progressive T wave inversion in which the T wave takes off from a concave or straight ST segment into a symmetrical and deeply inverted T wave; the angle between the ST segment and the downslope of the T wave is 60 to 90 degrees.[1-3]

In a study involving 180 patients, the ST-T segment abnormalities seen in leads V_2 and V_3 were also found in lead V_1 in 121 patients, in lead V_4 in 136 patients, and sometimes in leads V_5 and V_6 (Fig. 2–2B).[2]

NOTE: These ECG findings are seen in patients during the *pain-free* period. When patients experience chest pain, the findings are usually replaced by either ST segment elevation with positive T waves or ST segment depression with positive T waves.

UNSTABLE ANGINA

In de Zwaan's series of patients showing the ECG pattern of critical LAD stenosis, the severity of the unstable angina ranged from class III to class IV (angina at rest to angina during slight exercise). These complaints were present a mean of 6 days before admission.[2]

TIME FRAME FOR THE DEVELOPMENT OF THE TYPICAL ECG

The typical ECG findings of critical proximal LAD stenosis, described above, were present on admission in 60 percent of the 180 patients in de Zwaan's

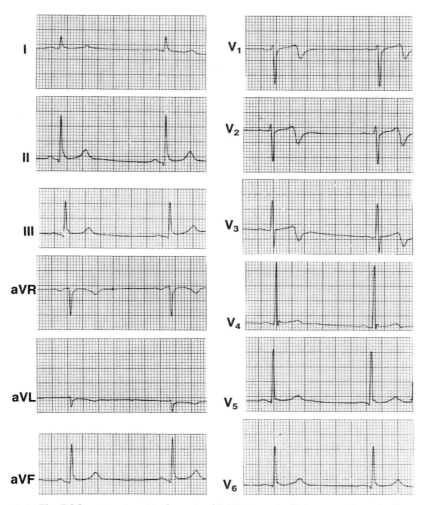

Figure 2–1. The ECG pattern in critical proximal LAD stenosis. This pattern is typically present when the patient is pain-free. The ST-T segment abnormalities are not limited to leads V_2 and V_3, but also frequently present in leads V_1, V_4, and V_5.

series.[2] In the majority of the remainder of patients, the ECG abnormalities developed within 24 hours; Figure 2–2 illustrates such a sequence. In a few patients the delay from admission to appearance of the typical ECG pattern for critical proximal LAD stenosis was 2 to 5 days. The patients who had ECG signs at the time of admission had a longer duration of unstable angina and a higher incidence of collateral formation than did the patients whose ECG signs developed later.

TREATMENT

In the past, patients with the ECG findings described above have been diagnosed as having either nontransmural or subendocardial ischemia (in

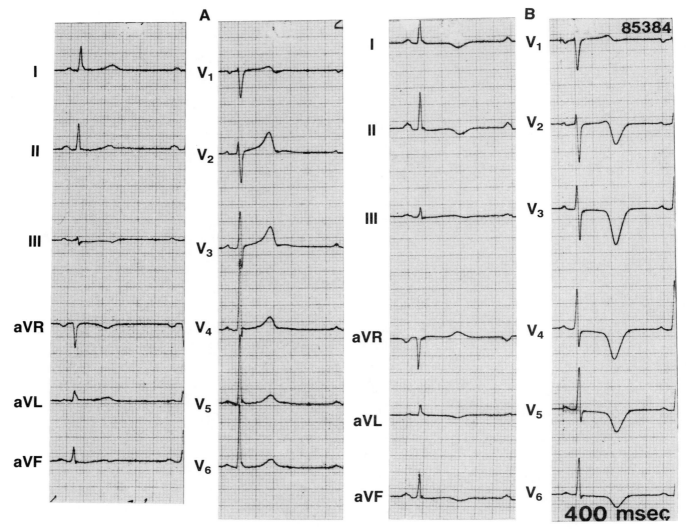

Figure 2–2. ECG changes reflecting critical proximal LAD stenosis. *(A)* The patient is admitted because of anginal pain. There is only a slight negativity at the end of the T waves in leads V_1 to V_3. Twelve hours later *(B)*, when pain has subsided, typical ST-T segment abnormalities with symmetrical deep inversion of the T wave are seen in leads V_2 to V_6.

the absence of enzyme changes) or non-Q wave (or subendocardial) infarction of the anterior wall in the presence of an enzyme elevation. However, in these patients significant myocardial infarction has not yet taken place, and emergency coronary angiography should be performed to identify candidates for early revascularization. Emergency angiography is justified in patients with unstable angina and this ECG pattern because the morbidity and mortality of cardiac catheterization and revascularization surgery are less than those of an extensive anterior wall myocardial infarction.

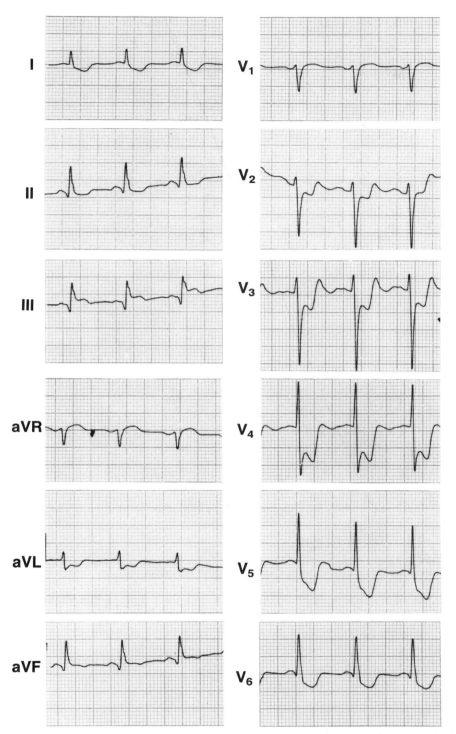

Figure 2–3. The ECG pattern of left mainstem disease. Note the ST segment elevation in leads V_1 and aVR and the ST segment depression in the remainder of the precordial leads and in leads I, II, and aVL. The patient had an old inferior myocardial infarction.

LEFT MAINSTEM AND THREE-VESSEL DISEASE

As discussed in Chapter 1, the size of the area at risk during myocardial infarction is reflected by the degree of ST segment changes and the number of leads in which these changes are present. Similarly, in patients with unstable angina, the extent of coronary artery disease can be diagnosed by certain ST segment changes. This frequently allows recognition of the high risk angina patient because of left mainstem or severe three-vessel disease.

ECG RECOGNITION

If there is ST segment elevation in leads V_1 and aVR plus ST segment depression in eight or more leads in a patient with unstable angina (Fig. 2–3), the chance of having severe left mainstem or three-vessel disease is very high (71 percent).[4]

In a study involving 125 patients with left mainstem disease, of the eight leads with ST depression, the most frequently involved leads were V_3 to V_5. Lead V_4 showed the greatest amount of ST depression (67 percent of patients).[5]

NOTE: Twenty-five percent of patients with as much as 91 to 99 percent occlusion of the left main coronary artery have a normal ECG when they are pain-free! It is therefore important to record the ECG *during* chest pain.

TREATMENT

It is important to recognize left mainstem and three-vessel disease and to revascularize the myocardium before infarction occurs. Especially when the characteristic ECG changes during anginal pain are accompanied by hypotension, emergency coronary catheterization and revascularization are required.

SUMMARY

Because of the life-preserving interventions now available, such as coronary bypass grafting and coronary angioplasty, early aggressive treatment is most desirable in patients with critical proximal LAD stenosis or severe left mainstem and three-vessel disease. It is now possible to recognize these conditions in patients with unstable angina and with no enzyme elevation because of their specific ECG findings. Critical proximal LAD stenosis is recognized because of progressive symmetrical T wave inversion in leads V_2 and V_3 with no loss of R wave. Severe left mainstem and three-vessel disease is recognized because of ST segment elevation in two leads (V_1 and aVR) and ST segment depression in eight other leads. Typically, whereas the ECG changes diagnostic of critical proximal LAD stenosis are best recognized *outside* the episode of anginal pain, the abnormalities suggestive of severe left mainstem or three-vessel disease are most marked on the ECG recorded *during* an attack of chest pain.

References

1. de Zwaan, C., Bar, F.W.H.M., and Wellens, H.J.J.: Characteristic electrocardiographic pattern indicating a critical stenosis high in left anterior descending coronary artery in patients admitted because of impending myocardial infarction. Am. Heart J. 103:730, 1982.
2. de Zwaan, C., Bar, F.W., Janssen, J.H.A., et al.: Angiographic and clinical characteristics of patients with unstable angina showing an ECG pattern indicating critical narrowing of the proximal LAD coronary artery. Am. Heart J. 117:657, 1989.
3. Wellens, H.J.J.: The electrocardiogram 80 years after Einthoven. J. Am. Coll. Cardiol. 7:484–491, 1986.
4. Gorgels, A.P., Vos, M.A., Bar, F.W., and Wellens, H.J.J.: An electrocardiographic pattern, characteristic for extensive myocardial ischemia. Circulation 78 (Suppl. II):1682, 1988.
5. Atie, J., Brugada, P., Smeets, J.L.R.M., et al.: Clinical presentation and prognosis of left main coronary disease in the 1990's. Eur. Heart J. 12:495, 1991.

CHAPTER

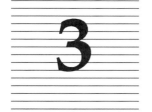

3

Wide QRS Tachycardia

EMERGENCY APPROACH

Do not panic when confronted with the broad QRS tachycardia. Obtain a 12-lead ECG.

IF HEMODYNAMICALLY UNSTABLE

1. Cardiovert.
2. Obtain a history.
3. Examine the pre- and postcardioversion ECGs to determine the etiology of the arrhythmia.

IF HEMODYNAMICALLY STABLE

1. Examine the patient for clinical signs of AV dissociation.
2. Systematically evaluate the 12-lead ECG.
3. Obtain a history.

IF VENTRICULAR TACHYCARDIA

1. Give procainamide 10 mg/kg body weight IV over 5 minutes unless the tachycardia is ischemia-related; then give lidocaine. If unsuccessful:
2. Cardiovert.
3. Examine the ECG during the ventricular tachycardia and the ECG during sinus rhythm to determine the etiology of the tachycardia.

IF SUPRAVENTRICULAR TACHYCARDIA WITH ABERRATION

1. Vagal stimulation; if unsuccessful:
2. Adenosine 6 mg by rapid IV bolus; if unsuccessful give 12 mg by rapid IV bolus; this dosage may be repeated once. If unavailable:
3. Verapamil 10 mg IV over 3 minutes; reduce to 5 mg if the patient is taking a beta blocker or is hypotensive. If unsuccessful:
4. Procainamide 10 mg/kg body weight IV over 5 minutes; if unsuccessful:
5. Cardiovert.
6. Examine supraventricular tachycardia and postconversion ECGs to determine mechanism.

IF IN DOUBT

Do not give verapamil; give IV procainamide.

IF IRREGULAR

Do not give digitalis or verapamil.
Give IV procainamide unless torsades de pointes is present (see Chapter 9).

INTRODUCTION

Because a drug given for the treatment of supraventricular tachycardia may be deleterious to a patient with ventricular tachycardia,[1, 2] the differential diagnosis in broad QRS tachycardia is critical. Errors are made because emergency care professionals wrongly consider ventricular tachycardia unlikely if the patient is hemodynamically stable,[3] and they are often unaware of the ECG findings that quickly and accurately distinguish ventricular tachycardia in more than 90 percent of cases. This chapter describes the mechanisms of aberrant ventricular conduction and the findings on physical examination and the ECG that help to differentiate aberrancy from ventricular ectopy.[4-6] Treatment and follow-up care also are discussed.

To arrive at the correct diagnosis it is important to understand the ECG features of ventricular tachycardia and supraventricular tachycardia with aberration and to search carefully for clues during physical examination.

CAUSES

The possible causes of wide QRS tachycardia are illustrated in Figure 3–1 and described here.

1. *Supraventricular tachycardia* with pre-existing or functional bundle branch block (BBB). This includes sinus tachycardia, atrial tachycardia, atrial flutter, atrial fibrillation, and AV nodal reentry tachycardia.
2. *Orthodromic circus movement tachycardia* using the AV node in the anterograde direction and an accessory pathway in the retrograde direction with pre-existing or functional bundle branch block
3. *Supraventricular tachycardia* with conduction over an accessory pathway
4. *Antidromic circus movement tachycardia* using an accessory pathway in the anterograde direction and the AV node or another accessory pathway in the retrograde direction
5. *AV reentry tachycardia* using a Mahaim fiber in the anterograde direction and the bundle of His or another accessory pathway in the retrograde direction
6. *Ventricular tachycardia*

PHYSICAL EVALUATION FOR AV DISSOCIATION

In addition to careful evaluation of the ECG, examination of the patient should include a search for physical signs of atrioventricular (AV) dissociation

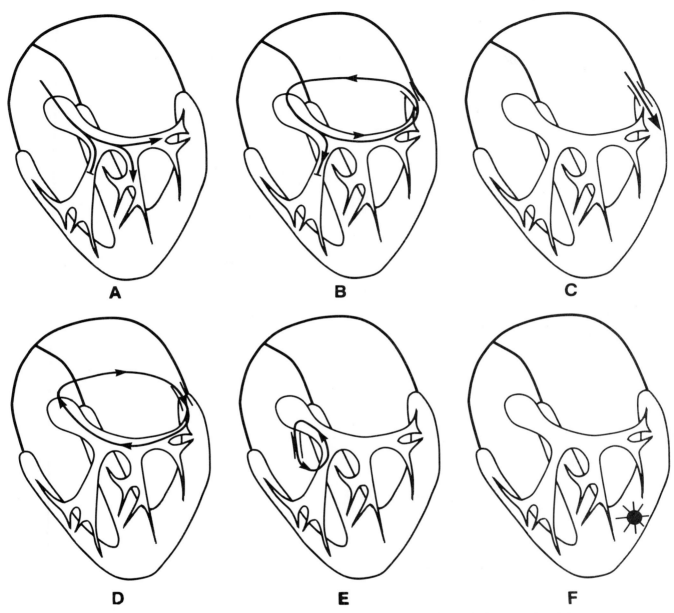

Figure 3–1. Illustration shows the different types of tachycardia with a wide QRS complex. *(A)* Supraventricular tachycardia (sinus tachycardia, atrial tachycardia, atrial flutter, atrial fibrillation), atrioventricular (AV) nodal reentry tachycardia, with pre-existent or tachycardia-related bundle branch block. *(B)* Circus movement tachycardia with AV conduction over the AV node and ventriculoatrial (VA) conduction over an accessory pathway in the presence of pre-existent or tachycardia-related bundle branch block. *(C)* Supraventricular tachycardia (sinus tachycardia, atrial tachycardia, atrial flutter, atrial fibrillation) with AV conduction over an accessory AV pathway. *(D)* Circus movement tachycardia with AV conduction over an accessory AV pathway and VA conduction over the AV node or (not shown) a second accessory AV pathway. *(E)* Tachycardia with anterograde conduction over a nodoventricular (Mahaim) fiber and retrograde conduction over the bundle of His or (not shown) a supraventricular tachycardia with AV conduction over a nodoventricular fiber. *(F)* Ventricular tachycardia.

(i.e., irregular cannon A waves in the jugular pulse, varying intensity of the first heart sound, and beat-to-beat changes in systolic blood pressure).[4, 7]

AV dissociation is present in approximately 50 percent of all ventricular tachycardias. The other 50 percent show some form of retrograde conduction to the atria. Thus, the finding of AV dissociation is an important diagnostic clue.

The physical signs of AV dissociation are:

1. Irregular cannon A waves in the jugular pulse
2. Varying intensity of the first heart sound
3. Beat-to-beat changes in systolic blood pressure

Any one of these three clues indicates AV dissociation. However, in the absence of such clues, ventricular tachycardia is still not ruled out; there remains the possibility of coexistent atrial fibrillation or ventriculoatrial conduction, in which case none of the signs of AV dissociation will be present. Theoretically, it is also possible for an AV junctional tachycardia with retrograde block to have AV dissociation; however, in view of the rarity of such a rhythm, AV dissociation remains a valuable diagnostic clue for ventricular tachycardia.

THE JUGULAR PULSE

In ventricular tachycardia with independent beating of atria and ventricles, the atria occasionally beat against closed AV valves because of simultaneous ventricular contraction. This causes a backflow of blood into the jugular vein, producing the so-called "cannon A waves." Inspection of the jugular vein reveals the characteristic occasional expansive pulsation.

VARYING INTENSITY OF THE FIRST HEART SOUND

The first heart sound marks the onset of ventricular systole and is caused by the closing of the mitral and tricuspid valves. Usually it is loudest at the apex, but at times it may be louder at the fourth left intercostal space.

During AV dissociation there is a beat-to-beat change in the loudness of the first heart sound due to the varying position of the AV valves at the time of ventricular contraction. Thus, the first heart sound varies in intensity during ventricular tachycardia and complete heart block, as well as during AV Wenckebach and atrial fibrillation.

CHANGES IN SYSTOLIC BLOOD PRESSURE

During AV dissociation ventricular filling from the atria varies, depending on the time lapse between atrial and ventricular contraction. These differences in ventricular filling lead to a beat-to-beat change in systolic stroke volume into the aorta, which in turn causes beat-to-beat changes in systolic blood pressure (Fig. 3–2). This sign of AV dissociation can easily be picked up at the bedside using the blood pressure recorder. Thus, a typical finding in ventricular tachycardia with AV dissociation is that the rhythm is regular, whereas the systolic blood pressure differs from beat to beat.

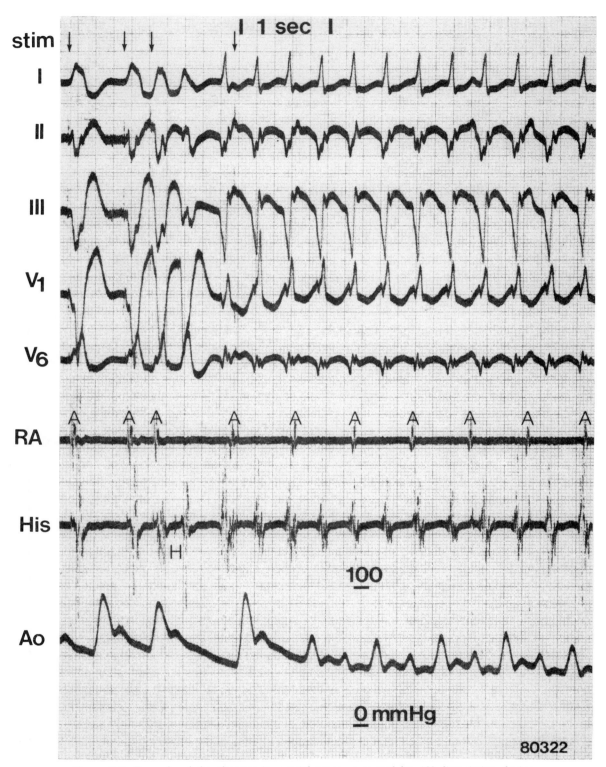

Figure 3–2. Example of the changes in arterial pressure caused by AV dissociation during ventricular tachycardia. Ventricular tachycardia was initiated in the catheterization laboratory by delivering two premature ventricular beats during ventricular pacing. Note in the aortic pressure tracing (Ao) that the systolic pressure changes relative to the timing of atrial contraction in relation to ventricular contraction. RA is a recording from inside the right atrium. The His bundle lead records the electrical activity of the heart at the site of the bundle of His.

MECHANISMS OF ABERRANT VENTRICULAR CONDUCTION

Aberrant ventricular conduction is a widening of the QRS due to delay or block in bundle branch or intramyocardial conduction secondary to:

1. Sudden shortening of the cycle length (phase 3 aberration)
2. Retrograde invasion into one of the bundle branches (retrograde concealed conduction), or
3. Slow rates (phase 4 aberration)

Delay or block in the right bundle branch is the most common cause of aberration because that bundle usually has the longest refractory period.[4, 8–10]

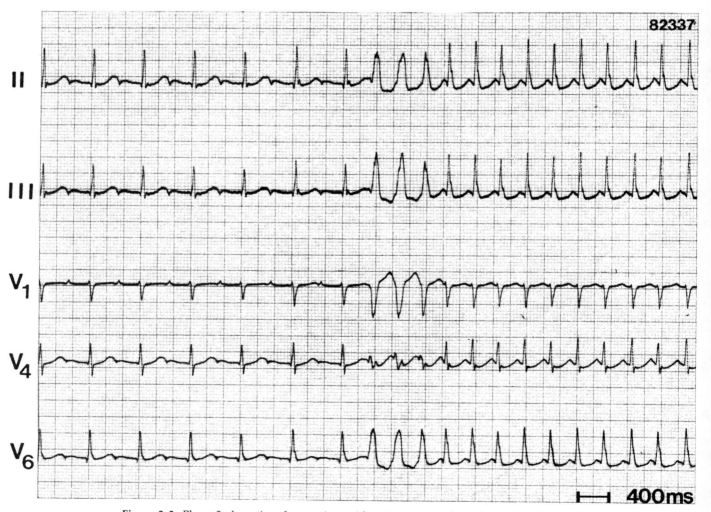

Figure 3–3. Phase 3 aberration. In a patient with a supraventricular tachycardia and 2:1 AV conduction (*left*) there is a sudden change to 1:1 AV conduction. This sudden increase in ventricular rate is accompanied by widening of the first three QRS complexes (LBBB). Note that the third QRS shows less widening than the first and second QRS complexes. This sequence is typical for phase 3 aberration.

Left bundle branch block (LBBB) aberration accounts for approximately one-third of cases with aberrant ventricular conduction.

PHASE 3 ABERRATION

Functional or physiological phase 3 aberration (bundle branch block) may occur in normal fibers if the impulse is premature enough to reach the cell when the membrane has not fully repolarized. This is the form of aberration that is commonly observed at the beginning of paroxysmal supraventricular tachycardia (PSVT) (Fig. 3–3).

Phase 3 aberration is also likely to occur following a long–short cycle sequence because the refractory period of the beat following the long cycle is prolonged. Figure 3–4 shows that different degrees of right bundle branch block (RBBB) are present, depending on the prematurity of the atrial premature beat.[10]

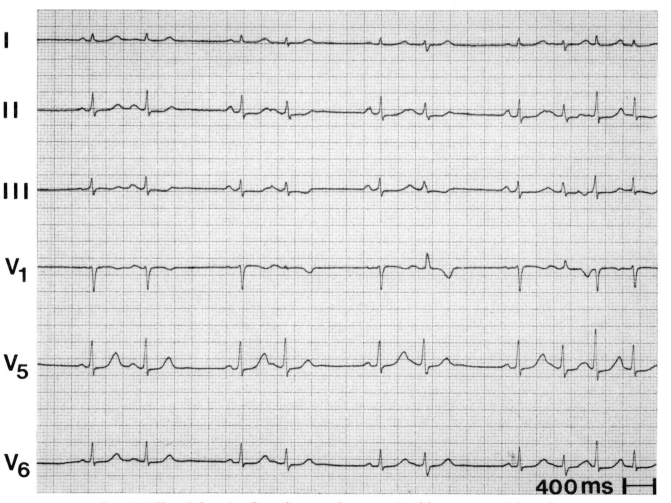

Figure 3–4. Phase 3 aberration. Depending upon the prematurity of the premature atrial complex (PAC), the QRS complex shows different degrees of aberrant conduction in the right bundle branch.

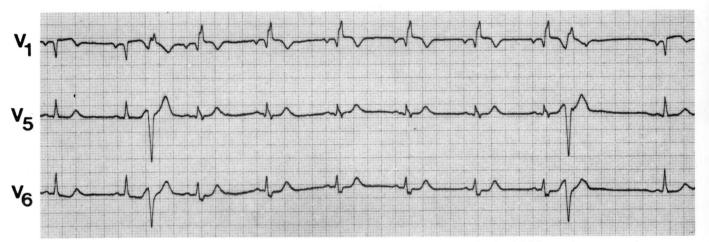

Figure 3–5. RBBB aberration due to retrograde concealed conduction. The third QRS complex is an interpolated premature ventricular contraction (PVC). This impulse, which originates in the left ventricle, is conducted in a retrograde fashion up the bundle branches. When the next sinus impulse reaches the bundle branches, only the left bundle branch has recovered excitability, and RBBB results. The impulse is conducted over the left bundle branch into the ventricles and in a retrograde fashion invades the right bundle branch, making it refractory again for the next sinus impulse. This mechanism continues until a new PVC is followed by a fully compensatory pause, allowing the right bundle branch time to recover.

CONCEALED RETROGRADE CONDUCTION

Although the mechanism at the onset of PSVT may be phase 3 aberration, the sustaining mechanism is often concealed retrograde conduction up one of the bundle branches. Figure 3–5 is an example of how, during sinus rhythm, RBBB aberration can be initiated by a premature ventricular complex (PVC). The mechanism of bundle branch block in the first sinus beat after the PVC is either phase 3 block of the right bundle or retrograde invasion of the PVC into the right bundle branch. This makes the right bundle branch refractory when the next supraventricular impulse passes through the AV node. The impulse is conducted down the left bundle branch and then in a retrograde direction up the right bundle branch. This mechanism is responsible for continuation of RBBB in subsequent conducted sinus beats. Retrograde invasion into the right bundle continues until disrupted by another PVC.

Retrograde concealed conduction into one of the bundle branches is a common mechanism of aberration during supraventricular tachycardias.[11]

PHASE 4 ABERRATION

Phase 4 aberration is bundle branch block and/or hemiblock that occurs only following a lengthening of the cardiac cycle. Conduction velocity is optimal

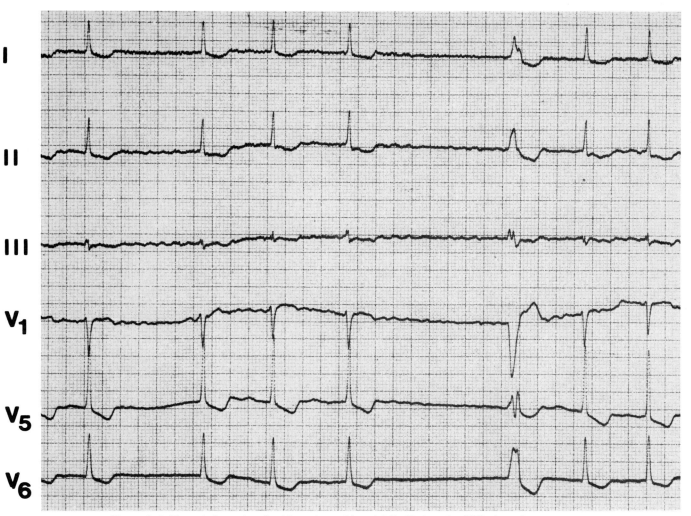

Figure 3–6. Phase 4 aberration. In this patient with atrial fibrillation, the QRS after a long pause shows an LBBB. This is caused by phase 4 block in the left bundle branch.

in fibers with a transmembrane potential of -90 mV, and it becomes slower when the membrane potential becomes less negative. During a long pause, the fibers of the His-Purkinje system are spontaneously depolarizing (becoming less and less negative), making it possible for block to occur with the impulse that terminates the pause. Phase 4 aberration also requires a shift in the threshold membrane potential to a less negative level and a change in membrane responsiveness. It is therefore seldom seen in normal hearts.

Figure 3–6 illustrates phase 4 LBBB aberration in a patient with atrial fibrillation. During a long cycle the membrane potential of the left bundle branch has become less and less negative, so that local delay or block takes place for the descending impulse.

SYSTEMATIC APPROACH TO WIDE QRS TACHYCARDIA

It is important to stay calm and approach the patient with a well-established, orderly, and correct protocol. Hemodynamic status is not a clue to the mechanism of the arrhythmia. Hemodynamic instability means only that you must cardiovert immediately, not that you are dealing with ventricular tachycardia.

WHEN THE PATIENT IS HEMODYNAMICALLY UNSTABLE

- Cardiovert.
- Stabilize.
- Evaluate systematically.
- Diagnose.

Once the hemodynamically stable patient has been cardioverted and stabilized, it is important to evaluate the preconversion 12-lead ECG for QRS configuration and signs of AV dissociation, QRS width, QRS axis, precordial concordance, and fusion beats in order to determine the mechanism of the tachycardia. Remember that every broad QRS tachycardia that is hemodynamically unstable is not necessarily ventricular tachycardia. If it is supraventricular tachycardia with aberration, there are important decisions to be made about the underlying mechanism. These are discussed in Chapter 4.

WHEN THE PATIENT IS HEMODYNAMICALLY STABLE

- Evaluate systematically.
- Diagnose.
- Treat.

A systematic approach consists of an evaluation of QRS configuration and physical and ECG signs of AV dissociation. Other helpful clues are QRS duration and axis. Precordial concordance, capture beats, and fusion beats are signs of ventricular tachycardia, but their occurrence is infrequent. Conditions besides hemodynamic status that cannot be used in the differential diagnosis are age and ventricular rate.

DIAGNOSTIC LEADS

To make a diagnosis on the basis of morphology, it is ideal to have a 12-lead ECG. It is absolutely necessary to record at least lead V_1; in many cases recordings of V_2 and V_6 are also necessary. If lead V_1 does not conclusively demonstrate ventricular tachycardia: (1) in the V_1-positive configuration, lead V_6 is needed; (2) in the V_1-negative configuration, leads V_2 and V_6 are needed.

If your ECG recording system does not have the capability for recording simultaneous leads, pay special attention to leads V_1, V_2, and V_6 for morphological clues and to leads I and II for axis.

QRS CONFIGURATION IN ABERRANT VENTRICULAR CONDUCTION

Aberrant ventricular conduction is either RBBB and/or hemiblock, or LBBB. The achievement of a correct diagnosis is dependent on the ability of the examiner to recognize the typical ECG patterns of bundle branch block versus that of ventricular tachycardia.

RIGHT BUNDLE BRANCH BLOCK ABERRATION

RBBB aberration is recognized because of a triphasic rSR' pattern in lead V_1 and a triphasic qRS pattern in lead V_6 (Fig. 3–7).[4, 12] In lead V_1 the initial r wave reflects normal septal activation; the S wave reflects left ventricular activation; and the R' wave reflects late activation of the right ventricle. In V_6 the narrow little q wave reflects normal septal activation. Lead V_6 shows an R/S ratio of more than 1 in RBBB aberration. A typical example of RBBB aberration during supraventricular tachycardia is shown in Figure 3–8.

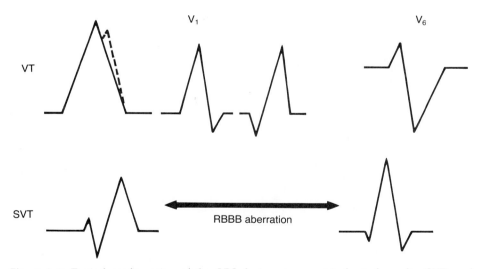

Figure 3–7. Typical configuration of the QRS during supraventricular tachycardia (SVT) and ventricular tachycardia (VT) in leads V_1 and V_6 when V_1 is positive. In lead V_1 a triphasic (rSR') pattern supports a diagnosis of supraventricular tachycardia; a monophasic or biphasic pattern supports a diagnosis of ventricular tachycardia. In lead V_6, a triphasic (qRS) pattern with R/S ratio >1 supports a diagnosis of supraventricular tachycardia; a deep S wave (R/S ratio < 1) supports a diagnosis of ventricular tachycardia.

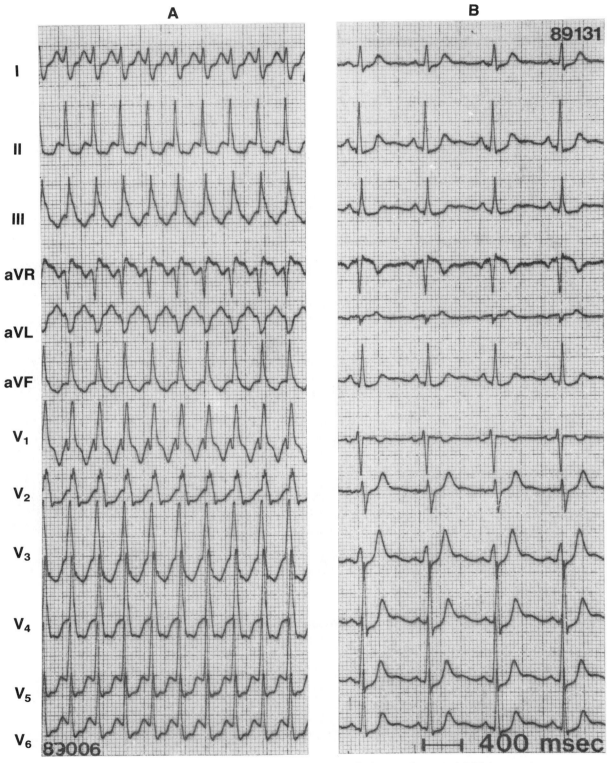

Figure 3–8. Supraventricular tachycardia with RBBB *(panel A)*. Note the typical QRS features in leads V₁ and V₆. *Panel B* shows sinus rhythm in the same patient.

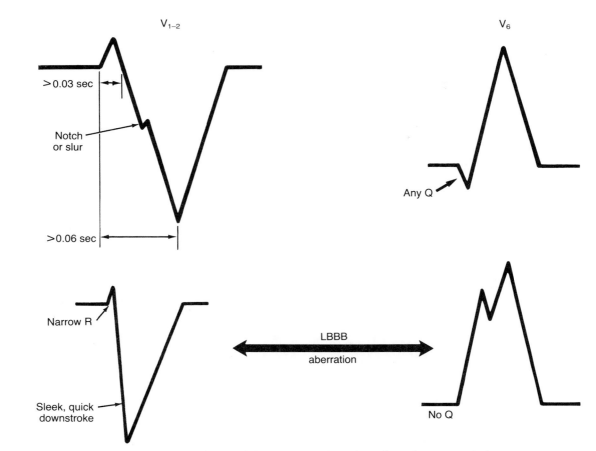

Figure 3–9. Typical configuration of the QRS during ventricular tachycardia and supraventricular tachycardia (SVT) in leads V_1, V_2, and V_6 when V_1 is predominantly negative. In leads V_1 and V_2, a narrow r and a clean, swift downstroke support a diagnosis of supraventricular tachycardia; a broad r, slurred downstroke, and/or delayed S nadir support a diagnosis of ventricular tachycardia. In lead V_6 any Q wave supports a diagnosis of ventricular tachycardia.

LEFT BUNDLE BRANCH BLOCK ABERRATION

A diagnosis of LBBB aberration is made in leads V_1 and V_2. If an r wave is present in either lead V_1 or V_2, it is narrow (less than 0.04 sec) in LBBB aberration, and the downstroke of the S wave is clean and swift (no slurs or notches). Because of the narrow r and/or the clean downstroke, the distance from the beginning of the QRS to the nadir of the S wave is 0.06 sec or less. Figure 3–9 schematically shows the typical pattern seen in LBBB aberration. A clinical example is given in Figure 3–10.

QRS CONFIGURATION IN VENTRICULAR TACHYCARDIA

V_1-POSITIVE

Figure 3–7 illustrates the distinguishing features of ventricular tachycardia as compared with those of supraventricular tachycardia with aberration

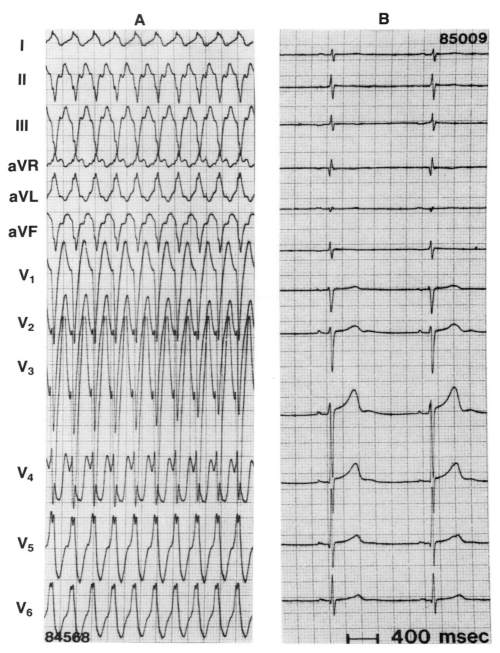

Figure 3–10. Supraventricular tachycardia with LBBB *(panel A)*. Note the typical QRS features in leads V_1 and V_2 (swift, clean downstroke, early S nadir, and the absence of a q in lead V_6). *Panel B* is from the same patient during sinus rhythm.

when there is a V_1-positive morphology. In lead V_1, a monophasic or biphasic pattern supports ventricular tachycardia, whereas a triphasic pattern (rSR′) favors supraventricular tachycardia (RBBB aberration). In lead V_6, a deep S (R/S ratio of <1) or QS indicates ventricular tachycardia, whereas a triphasic pattern (qRS) is suggestive for supraventricular tachycardia. In Figure 3–11, a diagnosis of ventricular tachycardia is made because of the monophasic R wave in lead V_1 and the deep S wave in lead V_6.[4, 12]

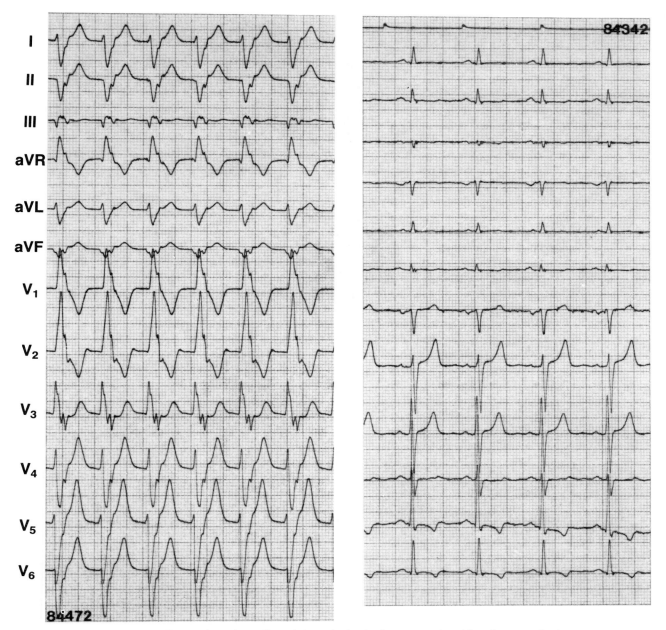

Figure 3–11. Ventricular tachycardia and sinus rhythm in the same patient. Note the monophasic R wave in lead V_1 and the deep S wave in lead V_6, signs of ventricular tachycardia. The northwest axis is also a helpful clue.

RABBIT EAR SIGN

When there are two positive peaks in lead V_1, ventricular ectopy is very likely if the left peak is the taller (Fig. 3–7, with dotted line). This is known as the "rabbit ear sign."[13] A taller right rabbit ear is of no help in distinguishing ventricular ectopy from aberration. In such a case the correct diagnosis should be made by evaluating V_6 or by noting signs of AV dissociation.

V_1-NEGATIVE

There are four morphological ECG signs found in leads V_1, V_2, and V_6 that are individually highly predictive of ventricular tachycardia.[5] They are:

1. A broad R of 0.04 sec or more in lead V_1 or V_2[5, 14, 15]
2. A slurred or notched S downstroke in lead V_1 or V_2
3. A distance of 0.07 sec or more from the onset of the ventricular complex to the nadir of the QS or S in lead V_1 or V_2
4. Any Q in lead V_6

In supraventricular tachycardia with LBBB aberration, if there is an r wave it is narrow and sharp in lead V_1 and/or V_2, and the S wave has a clean, swift downstroke in those leads.

The diagnostic morphological clues in lead V_6 are different for V_1-positive and V_1-negative broad QRS tachycardias. For example, a Q wave in lead V_6 could mean either ventricular tachycardia or supraventricular tachycardia, depending on the polarity of the total QRS complex in lead V_1. If V_1 is positive, a little q (<0.04 sec) in lead V_6 suggests supraventricular tachycardia, especially in the presence of an R/S ratio of >1; however, if lead V_1 is negative it indicates ventricular tachycardia.

Figure 3–9 illustrates the four distinguishing features of ventricular tachycardia compared with supraventricular tachycardia when there is a V_1-negative morphology. An example is given in Figure 3–12, where all four features are present.

It is important to use both leads V_1 and V_2 in this type of broad QRS tachycardia, since initial forces may be isoelectric in lead V_1, leading to misclassification. When lead V_1 has a supraventricular tachycardia morphology (narrow r and clean downstroke), it is especially important to look at leads V_2 and V_6 before making a diagnosis of supraventricular tachycardia. Additionally, measurement of the distance to the nadir of the S wave is sometimes not possible because of the depth of the S wave going off the graph paper.

Limitations. The limitations associated with these criteria for the differential diagnosis in V_1-negative broad QRS tachycardia include:

1. The rare case of LBBB in supraventricular tachycardia having the same morphology as ventricular tachycardia (broad R, slurred downstroke, etc., in leads V_1 and/or V_2). This may be found in patients with pre-existent LBBB and severe fibrotic disease of the left ventricle. In such a situation a comparison of the sinus rhythm tracing with that of the tachycardia will allow the correct diagnosis.

2. Antidromic circus movement tachycardia with anterograde conduction over an accessory pathway inserting in the right ventricle. Such a

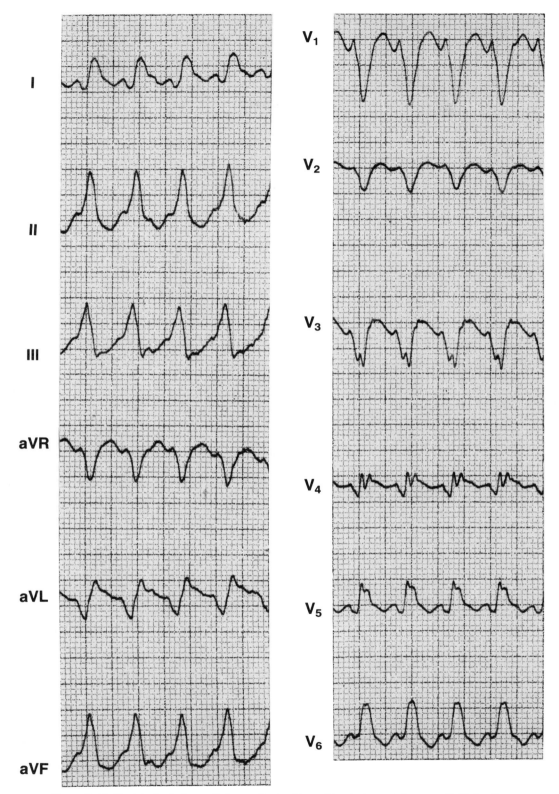

Figure 3–12. Ventricular tachycardia in a patient with an old anterior septal myocardial infarction. Note in lead V_1 the wide R wave and the prolonged interval between the beginning of the QRS to the nadir of the S wave. A qR pattern is present in lead V_6.

mechanism produces a tachycardia identical in morphology to the V_1-negative ventricular tachycardia.

3. The use of antiarrhythmic drugs that cause slow conduction, such as class IA (procainamide, quinidine, disopyramide) or class IC (encainide, flecainide, propafenone), may broaden the R wave and produce a delayed S nadir in lead V_1 or V_2.

ATRIAL ACTIVITY DURING VENTRICULAR TACHYCARDIA

One-half of all cases of ventricular tachycardia have AV dissociation; a few of the remainder have atrial fibrillation, and the rest have some form of retrograde conduction to the atria.[6] This may be 1:1 or 2:1 retrograde conduction or some form of retrograde Wenckebach; Figure 3–13 illustrates ventricular tachycardia with 7:6 retrograde Wenckebach conduction.

ECG RECOGNITION OF AV DISSOCIATION

Independent beating of atria and ventricles is the hallmark of ventricular tachycardia, and it can be recognized on the ECG when regular independent P waves are seen (Fig. 3–14). Such a finding is a very strong diagnostic sign of ventricular tachycardia. P wave identification may, however, be difficult or impossible, because T waves or terminal or initial parts of the ventricular complex may resemble P waves, leading to a misdiagnosis of supraventricular tachycardia. Because of this, the evaluation of QRS morphology and a physical examination for AV dissociation are faster and more reliable methods than is a search for P waves.

OTHER DIAGNOSTIC CLUES

QRS WIDTH

A QRS of 0.14 sec or more favors a diagnosis of ventricular tachycardia, especially in V_1-positive type tachycardia. When lead V_1 is negative, the QRS can be greater than 0.14 sec in both ventricular tachycardia and LBBB aberration because a QRS of this duration is not uncommon in a fibrotic heart during LBBB. Other exceptions to this rule are (1) supraventricular tachycardia in the patient using antiarrhythmic drugs that slow conduction, (2) pre-existing bundle branch block or (3) tachycardias with atrioventricular conduction over an accessory pathway. On the other hand, a ventricular tachycardia in digitalis toxicity may have a QRS duration of less than 0.14 sec because of its origin in one of the bundle branches (see Chapter 8 on digitalis intoxication).

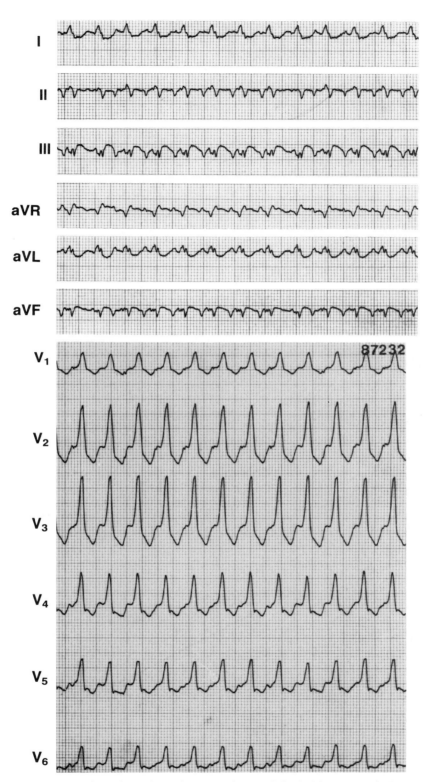

Figure 3–13. Ventricular tachycardia with retrograde Wenckebach. The retrograde P waves are nicely seen in leads II, III, and aVF. Note the lengthening RP intervals until a P wave is not conducted. The precordial leads show a positive concordant pattern.

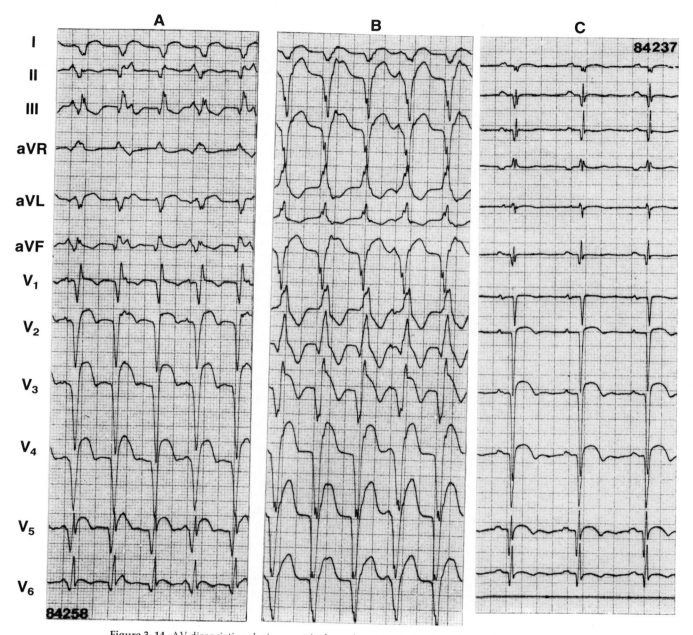

Figure 3–14. AV dissociation during ventricular tachycardia. In both *panels A* and *B,* independent P waves are visible throughout the tracing (best seen in leads II, III, and aVF). The ventricular tachycardia shown in *panels A* and *B* was recorded in a patient with an old extensive anterior wall myocardial infarction *(panel C).*

QRS AXIS IN THE FRONTAL PLANE

An abnormal axis is a strong indicator for ventricular tachycardia. This is especially true of an axis in the northwest quadrant (-90 degrees to ±180 degrees). In patients with prior myocardial infarction, an abnormal axis during ventricular tachycardia is quite common. Idiopathic ventricular tachycardia, however, frequently has a normal QRS axis.[16]

NARROW BEATS DURING WIDE QRS TACHYCARDIA

There are three mechanisms for a smaller beat during ventricular tachycardia: (1) a conducted sinus beat leading to capture or fusion, (2) an echo beat, and (3) another ventricular focus firing simultaneously or nearly so in the other ventricle.

Capture Beats or Fusion Beats

Occasionally during ventricular tachycardia one may observe a capture beat or a fusion beat. When a sinus impulse is conducted to the ventricles during ventricular tachycardia, it may either activate the ventricles entirely (capture) or activate the ventricles at the same time as the ventricular ectopic impulse (fusion); both circumstances result in a beat that is narrower than the complexes of the ventricular tachycardia. Figure 3–15 demonstrates ventricular fusion beats during ventricular tachycardia.

Echo Beats

During ventricular tachycardia it is possible for the impulse to enter the bundle branch system from a retrograde direction and be conducted back to the AV node to produce an atrial echo beat, which on return to the ventricle produces a narrow QRS complex (a reciprocal beat). In Figure 3–16 the three ventricular beats at the beginning of the tracing show retrograde conduction to the atria with progressive lengthening of the RP or ventriculoatrial (V-A) interval; this is best seen in leads II and III in this particular figure. This is followed by reentry in the AV node and return to the ventricle.

Two Ventricular Ectopic Foci

A narrower beat during ventricular tachycardia may also be produced when fusion occurs between the impulse responsible for ventricular tachycardia and a ventricular ectopic impulse arising in the other ventricle.

It is important to understand that a narrower beat during a wide QRS tachycardia is not always an indication of ventricular tachycardia, because in addition to the conditions already mentioned it may occur during supraventricular tachycardia with bundle branch block and PVCs arising in the ventricle having the bundle branch block. It may also happen during atrial fibrillation in the patient with an accessory AV pathway. In this case, it is the result of conduction of an occasional impulse down the AV node/bundle of His axis.

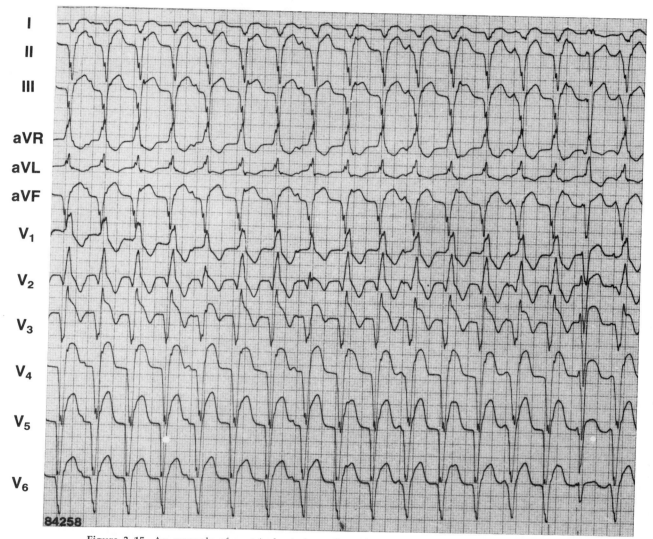

Figure 3–15. An example of ventricular tachycardia with ventricular fusion beats. The fifth, eighth, and sixteenth QRS complexes are narrower when compared with the other QRS complexes because of fusion between a ventricular ectopic complex and a conducted supraventricular beat.

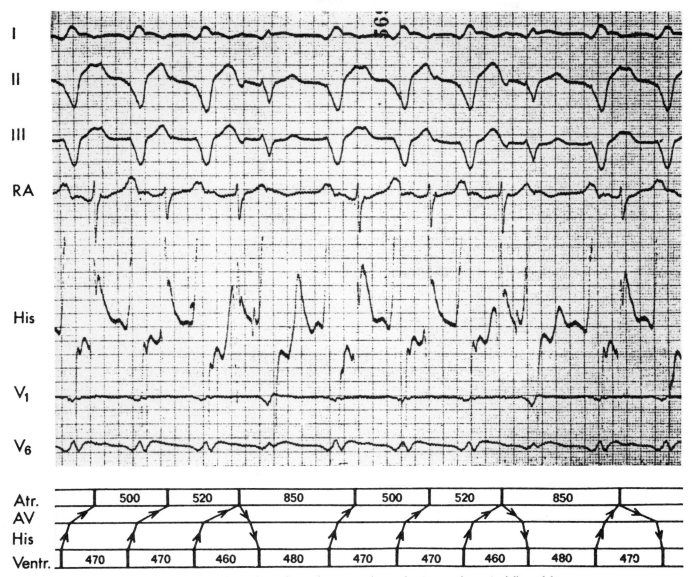

Figure 3–16. Ventricular tachycardia with retrograde conduction to the atria followed by an echo (or reciprocal) ventricular beat. Note the progressive lengthening of the RP interval after the first three ventricular ectopic beats. This is followed by a retrograde P wave and a ventricular "echo." That is, the retrograde P wave is conducted back down the AV node to the ventricles, producing a narrow QRS. The same sequence is repeated thereafter. To facilitate recognition of these phenomena, both right atrial (RA) and His bundle recordings are shown.

CONCORDANT PRECORDIAL PATTERN

A totally negative precordial pattern, as seen in Figure 3–17, is always
ventricular tachycardia because antidromic circus movement tachycardia
never has negative precordial concordance. This is because there is no

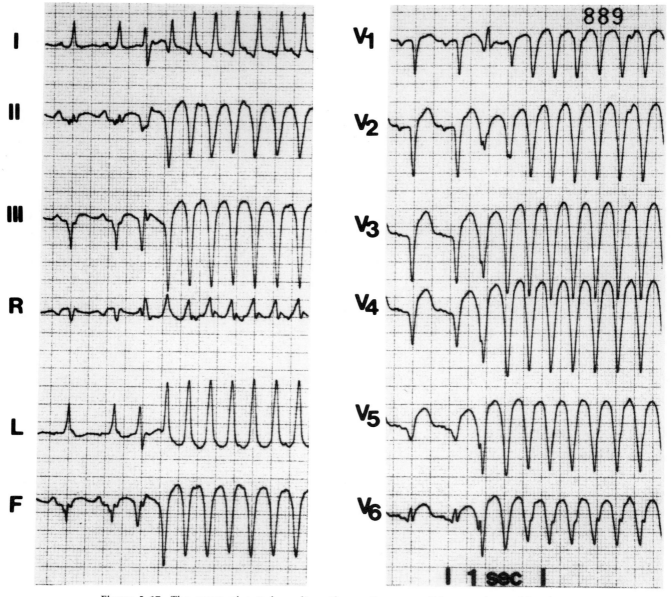

Figure 3–17. The onset of a tachycardia with negative precordial concordance. Negative
precordial concordance indicates ventricular tachycardia, since such a pattern does not occur
during anterograde conduction over an accessory pathway.

accessory pathway location where anterograde conduction over that structure leads to completely negative QRS complexes in all precordial leads.

On the other hand, a wide QRS tachycardia in which the QRS complexes are positive in all precordial leads may occur during ventricular tachycardia originating in the posterior wall of the left ventricle (Fig. 3–13) and also during a tachycardia using a left posterior accessory pathway for AV conduction. Figure 3–18 is an example of atrial flutter with 2:1 conduction over a left free wall accessory pathway, resulting in a positive precordial concordant pattern.

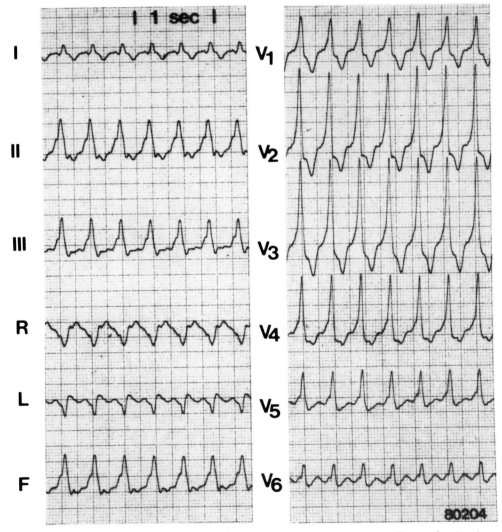

Figure 3–18. Broad QRS tachycardia with positive precordial concordance. The mechanism is atrial flutter with 2:1 conduction over a left-sided accessory pathway.

EMERGENCY TREATMENT

WHEN IN DOUBT

When a patient presents with a broad QRS tachycardia, diagnostic errors can be avoided by staying calm and using a systematic approach.

1. If the patient is in poor hemodynamic condition, cardiovert; otherwise, follow the diagnostic steps that will differentiate a supraventricular from a ventricular origin of the tachycardia (p. 46).

2. When in doubt about the origin of the tachycardia, *do not use verapamil;* use intravenous procainamide instead. One study observed a 44 percent incidence (11 of 25 patients) of severe hemodynamic deterioration when intravenous verapamil (5–10 mg) was administered during ventricular tachycardia, necessitating immediate cardioversion.[1] Hypotension with resulting ischemia may render the arrhythmia impossible to cardiovert.

Procainamide has advantages in both ventricular tachycardia and supraventricular tachycardia. It prolongs not only the refractory period of the ventricle but also that of an accessory AV pathway and the retrograde fast AV nodal pathway. Procainamide, therefore, may terminate ventricular tachycardia, circus movement tachycardia using an accessory pathway, and the common form of AV nodal reentry.

WHEN VENTRICULAR TACHYCARDIA IS THE DIAGNOSIS

1. Give IV procainamide 10 mg/kg body weight over 5 minutes; this prolongs the refractory period and slows conduction in the ventricle.

2. Use lidocaine only if acute myocardial ischemia (as in acute myocardial infarction) is considered to be the cause of the ventricular tachycardia.[17]

3. If antiarrhythmic drug therapy is unsuccessful, cardiovert.

WHEN SUPRAVENTRICULAR TACHYCARDIA IS THE DIAGNOSIS
(See also Chapter 4)

1. Use vagal stimulation to prolong the refractory period of the AV node. A good vagal maneuver in prehospital emergencies is to ask the patient to cough; other vagal maneuvers include carotid sinus massage, gagging, Valsalva maneuver, Trendelenburg position, squatting, and facial immersion in cold water. If unsuccessful:

2. Give adenosine[18] 6 mg IV over 1 to 2 seconds; if unsuccessful give 12 mg IV over 1 to 2 seconds and repeat 12-mg dosage if necessary. If adenosine is not available:

3. Give verapamil 10 mg IV in 3 minutes to block conduction in the AV node; reduce to 5 mg if the patient is taking a beta-blocking agent or is hypotensive. If unsuccessful:

4. Give IV procainamide 10 mg/kg body weight over 5 minutes. This may lead to block of the retrograde AV nodal pathway if the mechanism is

AV nodal reentry tachycardia; it may lead to retrograde block of the accessory pathway if the mechanism is circus movement tachycardia. Procainamide also prolongs the anterograde refractory period of an accessory AV pathway, thereby reducing the ventricular rate when the mechanism of the broad QRS tachycardia is atrial fibrillation with conduction over an accessory pathway. If unsuccessful:

    5. Cardiovert.

FOLLOW-UP CARE

WHEN CARDIOVERSION WAS THE FIRST THERAPEUTIC RESPONSE

    1. Obtain a postcardioversion 12-lead ECG.

    2. Carefully evaluate the pre- and postconversion tracings to determine the site of origin and (if possible) the pathway of the tachycardia. Examine the tracing during sinus rhythm for:

- Myocardial infarction, which makes ventricular tachycardia the most likely diagnosis
- Delta waves. Pre-excitation suggests that the mechanism of a wide QRS during supraventricular tachycardia is either circus movement tachycardia with bundle branch block or AV conduction over an accessory pathway.
- Bundle branch block. In cases of pre-existing bundle branch block, carefully compare the QRS during sinus rhythm with that during the tachycardia to diagnose ventricular tachycardia or supraventricular tachycardia with aberrant ventricular conduction. In supraventricular tachycardia with pre-existing bundle branch block, the QRS complex is often identical to that of the sinus rhythm.

    3. Take a careful history in order to establish the absence or presence of heart disease. Inquire as to how the arrhythmia was tolerated and events that may have triggered the episode, which may be prevented in the future. The answers to such questions are important because they help to determine the significance and prognosis of the attacks of tachycardia, and they help to determine the most appropriate therapy. Thus the patient who has had a sustained episode of a tachycardia should be asked:

- Have you had heart disease?
- Have you had tachycardia before? If so,
- At what age was the onset? (If the tachycardia was experienced initially at a young age, it is more likely to be supraventricular tachycardia than ventricular tachycardia.)
- How often does the tachycardia occur and how long does it last?
- Is there anything in particular that seems to trigger the onset of the tachycardia?
- Was there angina and/or dyspnea before or during the tachycardia?
- Did you feel faint or pass out during the tachycardia?

WHEN VENTRICULAR TACHYCARDIA IS THE DIAGNOSIS

Establish etiology of heart disease by the appropriate noninvasive and invasive tests and select long-term therapy accordingly.

WHEN SUPRAVENTRICULAR TACHYCARDIA IS THE DIAGNOSIS

Carefully study the preconversion tracings to determine the mechanism of the tachycardia. If an accessory pathway is involved, it is advisable to refer the patient to a cardiologist experienced in the study and management of tachycardias in the Wolff-Parkinson-White syndrome (see Chapter 4).

SIGNS AND SYMPTOMS THAT CANNOT BE USED

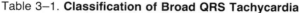

HEMODYNAMIC STATUS AND AGE

In the differential diagnosis of a broad QRS tachycardia, hemodynamic status and age should not be used as criteria, because ventricular tachycardia can occur at all ages, and some patients are hemodynamically stable in spite of ventricular tachycardia and hemodynamically compromised during supraventricular tachycardia. More emphasis should be placed on ECG findings in broad QRS tachycardia than on the patient's age or hemodynamic status.

Table 3–1. **Classification of Broad QRS Tachycardia**

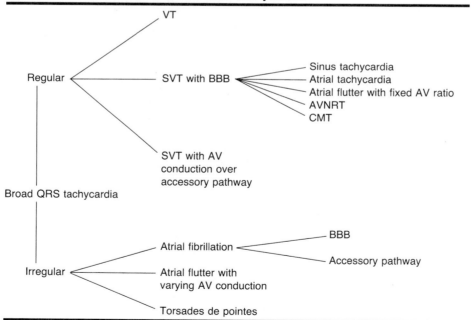

Abbreviations: AVNRT—AV nodal reentry tachycardia; CMT—circus movement tachycardia with AV conduction over the AV node and VA conduction over an accessory pathway; BBB—bundle branch block (functional or pathological); VT—ventricular tachycardia; SVT—supraventricular tachycardia.

VENTRICULAR RATE DURING THE TACHYCARDIA

Heart rate is not helpful in making the distinction between supraventricular tachycardia and ventricular tachycardia. Although supraventricular tachycardia tends to be faster than ventricular tachycardia, there is too much overlap to make this a useful criterion.

REGULARITY

Regular. A regular broad QRS tachycardia may be ventricular tachycardia, supraventricular tachycardia with bundle branch block, or supraventricular tachycardia with AV conduction over an accessory pathway.

Irregular. An irregular rhythm during a wide QRS tachycardia suggests bundle branch block during atrial fibrillation or atrial fibrillation with AV conduction over an accessory AV pathway. Occasionally, however, ventricular tachycardia, especially when drug-induced, may be very irregular (as in polymorphic ventricular tachycardia or torsades de pointes). Table 3–1 classifies broad QRS tachycardia according to regularity.

ANTIDROMIC CIRCUS MOVEMENT TACHYCARDIA

MECHANISM (See also Chapter 4)

Antidromic circus movement tachycardia (CMT) is based on a reentry circuit using an accessory pathway in the anterograde direction and the AV node or a second accessory pathway in the retrograde direction. Figure 3–19 illustrates this mechanism. The tachycardia that results is indistinguishable from ventricular tachycardia (Fig. 3–20).

EMERGENCY RESPONSE

1. Record a 12-lead ECG.
2. If hemodynamically unstable, cardiovert.
3. If hemodynamically stable, give IV procainamide 10 mg/kg over 5 minutes.
4. If a sinus rhythm is not restored, cardiovert.

ATRIAL FIBRILLATION WITH CONDUCTION OVER AN ACCESSORY PATHWAY

A broad QRS tachycardia that is irregular with a ventricular rate of more than 200 per minute and a QRS morphology identical to that of ventricular tachycardia should immediately arouse the suspicion of atrial fibrillation with conduction over an accessory pathway.[4]

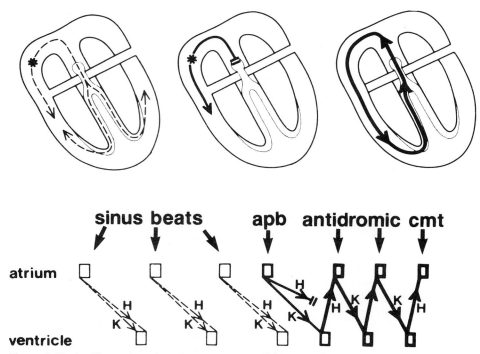

Figure 3–19. An illustration of initiation of antidromic circus movement tachycardia (cmt) by a premature atrial beat (apb). At a critical prematurity there is block in the AV node followed by AV conduction over the accessory pathway. The impulse then returns to the atria by way of the His bundle and AV node, and a CMT is established. Since the ventricle is activated by way of the accessory pathway, this tachycardia looks like ventricular tachycardia.

MECHANISM

In such a case, many of the atrial impulses are conducted to the ventricles over the accessory pathway (Fig. 3–21). The ventricular rate is dependent on the refractory period of the accessory pathway; the shorter the refractory period, the faster the ventricular rate. Apart from being rapid, this arrhythmia is irregular, and the QRS complexes resemble those of ventricular tachycardia in morphology because the accessory AV pathway inserts into the ventricle.

EMERGENCY RESPONSE

1. Record a 12-lead ECG.
2. If hemodynamically unstable, cardiovert.
3. If hemodynamically stable, give IV procainamide 10 mg/kg over 5 minutes (in Europe, ajmaline can be given, 1 mg/kg IV over 3 minutes).
4. If the ventricular rate does not slow with procainamide, cardiovert.

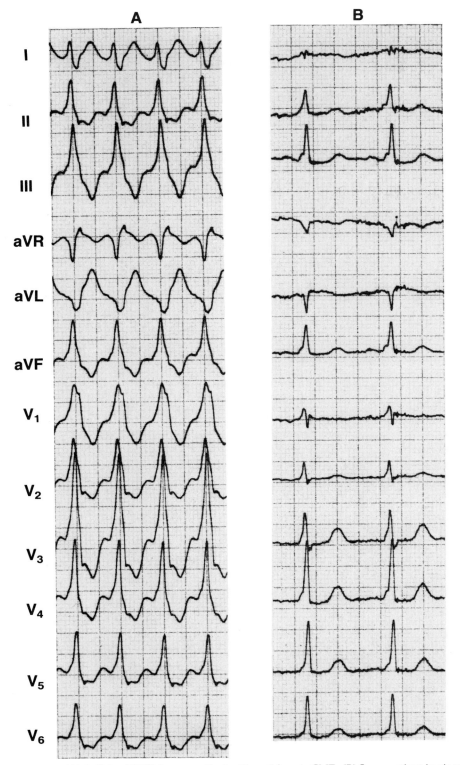

Figure 3–20. *(A)* A 12-lead ECG from a patient with antidromic CMT. *(B)* Same patient in sinus rhythm. Note that the delta wave polarity during sinus rhythm is the same as during tachycardia.

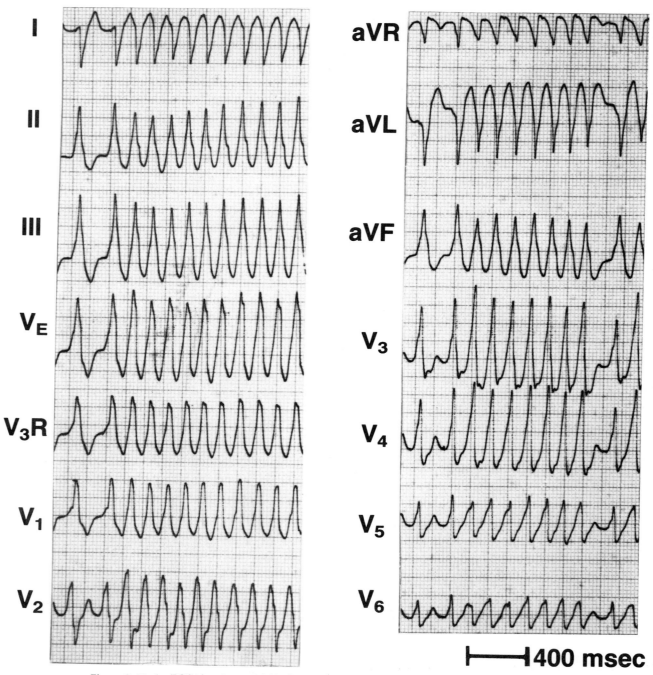

Figure 3–21. An ECG showing atrial fibrillation with AV conduction over an accessory pathway. The ventricular rate is determined by the anterograde refractory period of the accessory pathway. Note the rapid ventricular rate, broad QRS, and the irregular rhythm typical of this condition.

Patients with atrial fibrillation and an accessory pathway are at risk of dying suddenly because atrial fibrillation with a very high ventricular rate may deteriorate into ventricular fibrillation. Antiarrhythmic drugs are unlikely to control the problem.

5. If the ventricular rate slows and sinus rhythm is restored, the patient should be treated with drugs that prolong the refractory period of the accessory pathway and prevent the occurrence of premature beats that initiate atrial fibrillation.

Danger: Do not use digitalis or calcium channel blocker; such treatment may lead to a further increase in the ventricular rate. Digitalis may shorten the refractory period of the accessory pathway. A calcium blocking agent like verapamil may depress pump function, and subsequent sympathetic nervous system stimulation may lead to a further increase in ventricular rate.

Thus, emergency treatment using procainamide for the patient who is tolerating the arrhythmia also serves as a test. The clinical setting therefore offers a unique opportunity to evaluate the refractory period of the accessory pathway without electrophysiological studies. Procainamide or ajmaline (in Europe), when given intravenously, lengthens the refractory period in the accessory pathway; however, it does this to a different degree in individual patients.[19, 20] The response to these drugs during arial fibrillation therefore predicts whether the patient can be protected pharmacologically from rapid ventricular rates in the future. When, during atrial fibrillation with AV conduction over the accessory pathway, little or no slowing in ventricular rate can be obtained, the patient should be considered for radiofrequency or surgical ablation of the accessory pathway.

DIFFERENTIAL DIAGNOSIS WITH PRE-EXISTING BUNDLE BRANCH BLOCK

When there is a pre-existing bundle branch block, the differential diagnosis of a broad QRS tachycardia is made only after careful comparison of the QRS during the tachycardia with that during sinus rhythm. In Figure 3–22, the tachycardias in both panel A and panel B look like ventricular tachycardia when the morphological rules are applied. However, after careful comparison, it is clear that panel B represents supraventricular tachycardia because the complexes are identical to those seen during sinus rhythm.

SUPERIORITY OF PROCAINAMIDE OVER LIDOCAINE IN NONISCHEMIC VENTRICULAR TACHYCARDIA

In a randomized study involving a total of 56 episodes of sustained ventricular tachycardia occurring outside an episode of acute ischemia, procain-

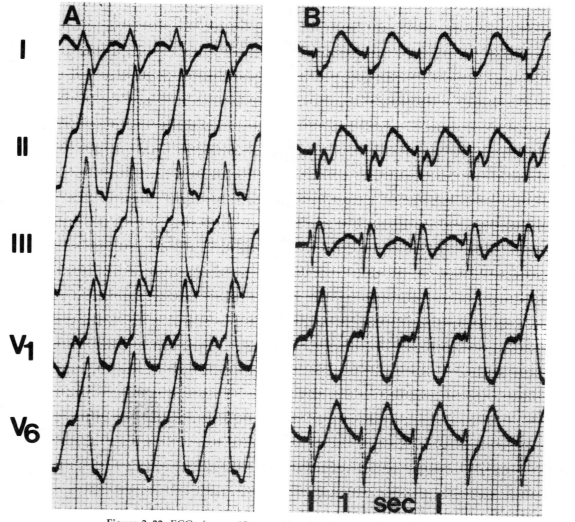

Figure 3–22. ECGs from a 15-year-old male who had complete correction of tetralogy of Fallot. *Panels A* and *B* show a tachycardia with a wide QRS complex. *Panel C* shows the QRS complex during sinus rhythm. Intracardiac recordings revealed that the tachycardia shown in *panel A* was of ventricular origin and that the one in *panel B* originated in the AV node. Note in *panel C* that pre-existent RBBB with left axis duration was present during sinus rhythm. This illustration was chosen to demonstrate that if a patient is admitted in tachycardia showing the recording as in *panel B*, the incorrect diagnosis of ventricular tachycardia probably would be made, using the criteria described. This shows the necessity of careful comparison with the ECG during sinus rhythm in patients with wide QRS during tachycardia.

amide was found to be clearly superior to lidocaine in terminating ventricular tachycardia. In this study, patients were randomly given either lidocaine 1.5 mg/kg in 3 minutes or procainamide 10 mg/kg in 5 minutes. When one drug failed to convert the ventricular tachycardia, the other drug was used after 20 minutes. Lidocaine terminated only four of 22 episodes of ventricular tachycardia, whereas procainamide terminated 24 of 32 episodes.[17]

SUMMARY

In the regular wide QRS tachycardia, the first task is to differentiate between ventricular tachycardia and supraventricular tachycardia with aberrant conduction (bundle branch block).

Certain morphological findings on the ECG can quickly and accurately pinpoint ventricular tachycardia in more than 90 percent of cases. When the tachycardia is V_1-positive, a diagnosis of RBBB aberration is supported by an rSR' pattern in lead V_1 or a qRS complex in lead V_6; ventricular tachycardia is very likely present when there is a monophasic or biphasic complex in lead V_1 or an R/S ratio of less than 1 in lead V_6 (the S wave is deeper than the R wave is tall).

When the tachycardia is V_1-negative, a diagnosis of LBBB aberration is supported when there are a sharp, narrow r and a smooth, quick downstroke to the S in lead V_1 and/or V_2; ventricular tachycardia is very likely when there is a fat R (>0.03 sec), a slurred or notched S downstroke, or a delayed S-nadir (>0.06 sec) in lead V_1 or V_2 or a Q in lead V_6.

Other indicators of ventricular tachycardia are AV dissociation (physical or ECG signs), a "northwest" QRS axis, QRS width greater than 0.14 sec, precordial concordance, fusion beats, and capture beats.

Apart from bundle branch block aberration, a wide QRS complex may occur in Wolff-Parkinson-White syndrome when an antidromic circus movement tachycardia is present or during atrial fibrillation, in which case the rhythm is irregular.

The emergency response to broad QRS tachycardia demands a calm, informed, and systematic approach. A 12-lead ECG is obtained and cardioversion performed if the patient is hemodynamically unstable. If stable, determine the type of tachycardia by systematically evaluating the 12-lead ECG, doing a physical examination, and obtaining a history.

In general, treatment for ventricular tachycardia is intravenous procainamide for nonischemic ventricular tachycardia and lidocaine for acute ischemic ventricular tachycardia. In supraventricular tachycardia with a regular rhythm, vagal maneuvers should be tried first. They may terminate the tachycardia or reveal the mechanism (such as atrial flutter); when tachycardia persists, adenosine, verapamil, or procainamide may be used. If irregular, procainamide should be used; if unsuccessful, electrical cardioversion should be employed.

References

1. Stewart, R.B., Bardy, G.H., and Greene, H.L.: Wide complex tachycardia: Misdiagnosis and outcome after emergent therapy. Ann. Intern. Med. 104:766–771, 1986.
2. Buxton, A.E., Marchlinski, F.E., Doherty, J.U., et al.: Hazards of intravenous verapamil for sustained ventricular tachycardia. Am. J. Cardiol. 59:1107–1110, 1987.
3. Dancy, M., Camm, A.J., and Ward, D.: Misdiagnosis of chronic recurrent ventricular tachycardia. Lancet 2:320–323, 1985.
4. Wellens, H.J.J., Bar, F.W.H.M., and Lie, K.I.: The value of the electrocardiogram in the differential diagnosis of a tachycardia with a widened QRS complex. Am. J. Med. 64:27, 1978.
5. Kindwall, E., Brown, J., and Josephson, M.E.: Electrocardiographic criteria for ventricular tachycardia in wide complex left bundle branch block morphology tachycardia. Am. J. Cardiol. 61:1279–1283, 1988.

6. Wellens, H.J.J., Bar, F.W., Brugada, P., and Farré, J.: The differentiation between ventricular tachycardia and supraventricular tachycardia with aberrant conduction: the value of the 12 lead electrocardiogram. In Wellens, H.J.J., and Kulbertus, H.E. (eds.): What's New in Electrocardiography? The Hague, 1981, Martinus Nijhoff, pp. 184–199.

7. Harvey, W.P., and Ronan, J.A.: Bedside diagnosis of arrhythmias. Prog. Cardiovasc. Dis. 8:419–431, 1966.

8. Lewis, R.: Paroxysmal tachycardia, the result of ectopic impulse formation. Heart 1:262, 1919.

9. Couax, F.J.L., and Ashman, R.: Auricular fibrillation with aberration simulating ventricular paroxysmal tachycardia. Am. Heart J. 34:366, 1957.

10. Moe, G.K., Mendez, C., and Han, J.: Aberrant AV impulse propagation in the dog heart: A study of functional bundle branch block. Circ. Res. 16:261, 1965.

11. Wellens, H.J.J., Ross, D.L., Farré, J., and Brugada, P.: Functional bundle branch block during supraventricular tachycardia in man: Observations on mechanisms and their incidence. In Zipes, D., and Jalife, J. (eds.): Cardiac Electrophysiology and Arrhythmias. New York, 1985, Grune and Stratton, pp. 435–441.

12. Marriott, H.J.L.: Differential diagnosis of supraventricular and ventricular tachycardia. Geriatrics 25:91, 1970.

13. Gozensky, C., and Thorne, D.: Rabbit ears: An aid in distinguishing ventricular ectopy from aberration. Heart Lung 3:634, 1975.

14. Rosenbaum, M.B.: Classification of ventricular extrasystoles according to form. J. Electrocardiol. 2:269, 1969.

15. Swanick, E.J., La Camera, F., and Marriott, H.J.L.: Morphologic features of right ventricular ectopic beats. Am. J. Cardiol. 30:888, 1972.

16. Coumel, P., Leclercq, J.F., Attuel, P., et al.: The QRS morphology in post-myocardial infarction ventricular tachycardia. A study in 100 tracings compared with 70 cases of idiopathic ventricular tachycardia. Eur. Heart J. 5:792–799, 1984.

17. Gorgels, A.P., van den Dool, A., Hofs, A., et al.: Procainamide is superior to lidocaine in terminating sustained ventricular tachycardia. Circulation 80 (Suppl II):2590, 1989.

18. Pinski, S.L., and Maloney, J.D.: Adenosine: A new drug for acute termination of supraventricular tachycardia. Cleve. Clin. J. Med. 57:383–388, 1990.

19. Wellens, H.J.J., Bar, F. W., Gorgels, A.P., et al.: Use of ajmaline in patients with Wolff-Parkinson-White syndrome to disclose a short refractory period of the accessory pathway. Am. J. Cardiol. 45:130, 1980.

20. Wellens, H.J.J., Braat, S., Brugada, P., et al.: Use of procainamide in patients with the Wolff-Parkinson-White syndrome to disclose a short refractory period of the accessory pathway. Am. J. Cardiol. 50:1087, 1982.

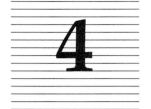

4

Narrow QRS Tachycardia

EMERGENCY APPROACH

Obtain a 12-lead ECG.
Assess the hemodynamic situation.

IF HEMODYNAMICALLY UNSTABLE

1. Cardiovert.
2. Obtain a history.
3. Record postconversion ECG.
4. Examine and compare pre- and postcardioversion ECGs to determine the type of supraventricular tachycardia, using a systematic approach.

IF HEMODYNAMICALLY STABLE

1. Look for the "frog sign" in the jugular pulse.
2. Perform vagal stimulation; if unsuccessful:
3. Give adenosine or verapamil:
   - *Adenosine* 6 mg as a rapid IV bolus; if unsuccessful increase dosage to 12 mg; this may be repeated.
   - *Verapamil* 10 mg IV over 3 minutes; reduce to 5 mg if the patient is taking a beta blocker or is hypotensive; if unsuccessful:
4. Give procainamide 10 mg/kg body weight over 5 minutes; if unsuccessful:
5. Perform electrical cardioversion.
6. Obtain a history.
7. Record a postconversion ECG.
8. Examine and compare the pre- and postconversion ECGs to determine the type of supraventricular tachycardia, using a systematic approach.

INTRODUCTION

Narrow QRS tachycardia is a cardiac rhythm with a rate faster than 100 beats per minute and a QRS duration of less than 0.12 sec. The narrow QRS indicates that atrioventricular (AV) conduction occurs via the AV node. The term "supraventricular tachycardia" is also used for this condition. However, during supraventricular tachycardia the QRS may be broad because of pre-existing bundle branch block, functional bundle branch block, or AV conduction over an accessory AV pathway. The patient with narrow QRS tachycardia usually seeks medical attention because of "palpitations," light-headedness, shortness of breath, or anxiety. Because of the paroxysmal character of supraventricular tachycardia, patients with this condition frequently have years of complaints before the cause is correctly diagnosed or before they even seek medical attention. It is therefore of extreme importance to obtain ECG documentation of the tachycardia so that the patient can receive the correct treatment. This chapter addresses causes, physical examination, anatomical substrate, mechanism, differential diagnosis, and treatment of narrow QRS tachycardias, and the effect of carotid sinus massage on supraventricular tachycardias.

CAUSES OF NARROW QRS TACHYCARDIA

1. Sinus tachycardia
2. Atrial tachycardia (nonparoxysmal and paroxysmal)
3. Atrial flutter
4. Atrial fibrillation
5. AV nodal reentry tachycardia
6. Orthodromic circus movement tachycardia

Figure 4–1 is a representation of the origin and mechanism of the three most common types of a regular supraventricular tachycardia: (A) atrial tachycardia, (B) AV nodal reentry tachycardia, and (C) circus movement tachycardia using an accessory pathway. This diagram illustrates the importance of evaluating P wave position and polarity when making the differential diagnosis in supraventricular tachycardia. The tachycardias illustrated in Figure 4–1 are usually paroxysmal, rarely permanent or incessant.

Nonparoxysmal atrial tachycardia caused by digitalis intoxication, another cardiac emergency, is discussed in Chapter 8.

Most of this chapter is devoted to the differential diagnosis of the most common causes of a regular narrow QRS tachycardia that may present as a cardiac emergency. They are AV nodal reentry tachycardia and orthodromic circus movement tachycardia.

SYSTEMATIC APPROACH

To arrive at the correct diagnosis it is important to:

1. Carefully search for clues during physical examination
2. Understand the mechanisms and ECG features of the different types of narrow QRS tachycardia
3. Meticulously evaluate the ECG during the tachycardia as compared with the sinus rhythm in the same leads
4. Evaluate the ECG during carotid sinus massage

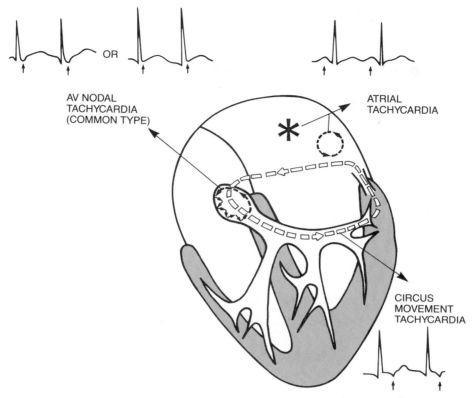

Figure 4–1. A representation of the sites of origin and mechanisms of paroxysmal supraventric- ular tachycardia as determined by the position and polarity of the P waves in relation to the QRS complex. In atrial tachycardia the P wave precedes the QRS; its polarity in lead III depends upon its location. In AV nodal reentry tachycardia the P wave is buried within the QRS or may distort the end of the QRS; that portion of the QRS is then negative in lead III. In circus movement tachycardia the P wave follows the QRS.

PHYSICAL EXAMINATION DURING SUPRAVENTRICULAR TACHYCARDIA

The physical findings in supraventricular tachycardia are summarized in Table 4–1. Careful physical examination during tachycardia can help to establish the origin of the arrhythmia. For example:

PULSE, BLOOD PRESSURE, AND FIRST HEART SOUND

In all types of regular supraventricular tachycardia, the pulse is regular and the blood pressure and the loudness of the first heart sound are constant.

In atrial fibrillation and atrial flutter with changing AV conduction and changing intervals between successive QRS complexes, the pulse, blood pressure, and loudness of the first heart sound vary.[1]

Table 4–1. **Clinical Findings and Blood Pressure Behavior in
Supraventricular Tachycardia**

Type of SVT	Pulse	Neck Vein Pulsation	Systolic Blood Pressure	Loudness of First Heart Sound
Sinus tachycardia	Regular	Normal	Constant	Constant
Atrial tachycardia	Regular	Normal	Constant	Constant
Atrial flutter	(a) Regular when 2:1 conduction; (b) irregular with variable conduction	Flutter waves	(a) Constant if regular pulse; (b) changing if irregular pulse	Constant
Atrial fibrillation	Irregular	Irregular pulsation	Changing	Changing
AV nodal tachycardia	Regular	"Frog" sign	Constant	Constant
Circus movement tachycardia	Regular	"Frog" sign	Constant	Constant

Data from Wellens, H.J.J., Brugada, P., and Bar, F.: Diagnosis and treatment of the regular tachycardia with a narrow QRS complex. In Kulbertus, H.E. (ed.): Medical Management of Cardiac Arrhythmias. Edinburgh, 1986, Churchill-Livingstone.

NECK VEINS

The pulsations in the neck veins often reveal the mechanism of the tachycardia.[2] For example:

Sinus tachycardia and atrial tachycardia are the only two supraventricular tachycardias that do not result in abnormal pulsations in the neck veins.
In atrial flutter there are flutter waves in the neck veins.
In atrial fibrillation there are irregular pulsations in the neck veins.

The Frog Sign. In AV nodal reentry tachycardia or circus movement tachycardia, the patient, and perhaps the family when questioned, may have noticed the *"frog sign."* That is, when the atria and ventricles are activated simultaneously, as in AV nodal reentry tachycardia, or when ventricular activation closely precedes atrial activation, as in circus movement tachycardia, the atria contract against closed AV valves, producing rapid, regular, expansive venous pulsations in the neck resembling the rhythmic puffing motion of a frog.

AV NODAL REENTRY TACHYCARDIA

ANATOMICAL SUBSTRATE

In patients with AV nodal reentry tachycardia, the arrhythmia is usually based upon reentry using two separate pathways within the AV node having different refractory periods and different conduction velocities. These two pathways are connected proximally (close to the atrium) and distally (close to the His bundle).

MECHANISM

In AV nodal reentry tachycardia, an impulse circulates within the AV node with activation of the ventricles from the anterograde path of the circuit and activation of the atrium from the retrograde path. There are two forms of AV nodal reentry tachycardia; their mechanisms are illustrated in Figure 4–2. In the common form (Fig. 4–2A), the slow intranodal pathway is the anterograde arm of the circuit and the fast pathway is the retrograde arm. In the rare form (Fig. 4–2B), the ventricles are activated via the fast pathway and the atria via the slow pathway. Both forms produce a typical ECG pattern.

Figure 4–2A illustrates the fact that the slow AV nodal pathway has a shorter refractory period than the fast pathway. Therefore, if a premature atrial complex (PAC) arrives at the proximal connection of the two pathways when the fast pathway is refractory and the slow pathway nonrefractory, it is conducted only over the slow pathway to the ventricles. At the distal site of the communication, the impulse not only activates the ventricles by way of the His-Purkinje system, but also crosses over and travels up the fast pathway to reenter the atria. This establishes a circulating wavefront within the AV node and results in simultaneous activation of atria and ventricles

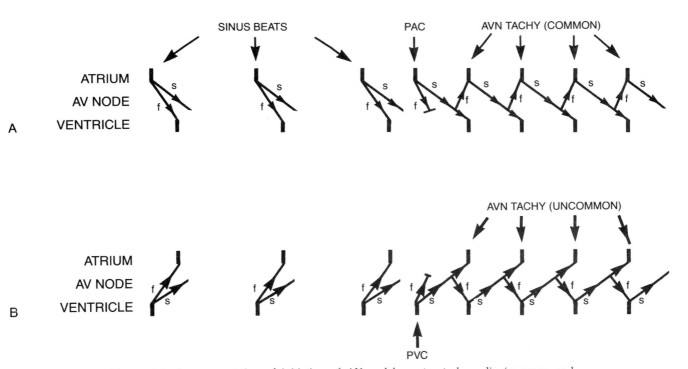

Figure 4–2. A representation of initiation of AV nodal reentry tachycardia (common and uncommon types). (A) Common type of AV nodal reentrant tachycardia. During sinus rhythm the impulse is conducted anterogradely through the AV node. A premature atrial complex (PAC) is blocked in the fast pathway, is conducted over the slow pathway to the ventricle, and returns to the atrium over the fast pathway. This establishes an intranodal circuit with simultaneous reentry into atria and ventricles, and it results in a retrograde P wave that is buried within or distorts the end of the QRS. (B) Uncommon type of AV nodal reentrant tachycardia. During a ventricular paced rhythm the impulse is conducted retrogradely through the AV node over the fast (f) pathway. A premature ventricular contraction (PVC) is blocked in the fast pathway, is conducted to the atrium over the slow (s) pathway, and returns to the ventricle by way of the fast pathway. This creates a circuit, with activation of the ventricle before activation of the atrium.

and the typical ECG pattern of the common form of AV nodal reentry tachycardia. Note that due to the slow anterograde and fast retrograde conduction, atrial activation and ventricular activation are simultaneous and the retrograde P waves are hidden within the QRS or occur during the end of the QRS, looking like a terminal R wave in lead V_1 (pseudo-right bundle branch block pattern) and an s wave in the inferior leads (II, III, aVF).

Figure 4–2B illustrates the initiation of AV nodal reentry tachycardia by a premature ventricular complex (PVC) during ventricular pacing. The initial portion of this illustration demonstrates retrograde conduction over the fast intranodal pathway. Following a PVC, the ventricular impulse is blocked in the fast pathway and conducted to the atria only via the slow pathway. The impulse then returns to the ventricles via the now nonrefractory fast pathway, and a reentry circuit is established for the uncommon form of AV nodal reentry tachycardia in which the anterograde limb of the circuit within the AV node is the fast pathway.

ECG RECOGNITION

- Fast, regular rhythm
- Paroxysmal
- QRS less than 0.12 sec
- P waves:

Common Form. P waves are usually hidden within the QRS, frequently in its terminal portion, resulting in pseudo-r waves in lead V_1 (a pseudo-right bundle branch block pattern) and pseudo-S waves in leads II, III, and aVF. Rarely, the P wave appears at the beginning of the QRS, resulting in pseudo-Q waves in leads II, III, and aVF.

Rare Form. P waves are negative in leads II, III, and aVF, and follow the QRS with an RP interval that is equal to or longer than the PR interval.

Recognition of AV nodal reentry tachycardia depends upon noting that the P waves are either totally hidden within the QRS or are distorting the terminal forces of the QRS. Therefore, recording the 12-lead ECG both during the tachycardia and during the sinus rhythm is important to facilitate recognition of the P wave during tachycardia. Because P waves are sometimes not seen in all leads, it is best to obtain recordings of all 12 leads. If this is not possible, one should at least strive to obtain five leads—I, II, III, V_1, and V_6. When the P waves are totally hidden within the QRS, this fact can be established by noting that the QRS is identical in shape in both the sinus rhythm and the tachycardia. When the P waves are distorting the end or beginning of the QRS, looking like terminal or initial forces of the QRS, they can be recognized by comparing the QRS during the tachycardia with that during sinus rhythm.

Figure 4–3 demonstrates how valuable the ECG during sinus rhythm can be in finding the P waves during the tachycardia. In comparing the QRS of the rhythm in Figure 4–3, P waves are seen during the tachycardia distorting the terminal QRS in leads II, III, and V_1, indicating the presence of AV nodal reentry tachycardia with simultaneous atrial and ventricular activation.

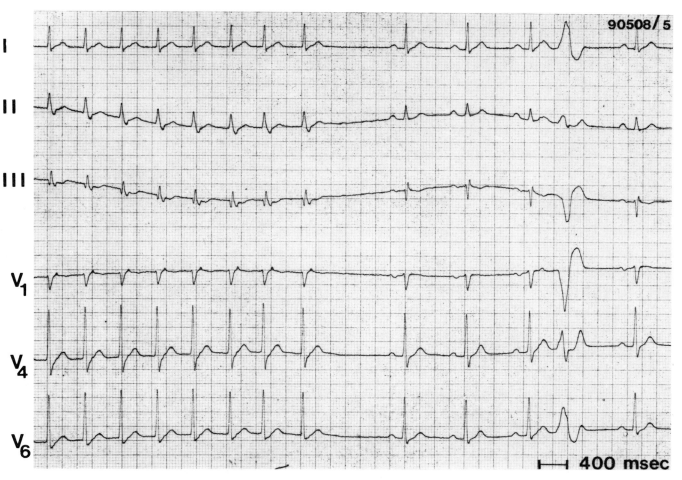

Figure 4–3. An example of the common type of AV nodal reentry tachycardia. The diagnosis is based on the position of the P waves during the tachycardia. Note that when compared with the sinus rhythm, the QRS of the tachycardia has a distortion of terminal forces in leads II, III, and V$_1$.

CLINICAL IMPLICATIONS

The tachycardia that results from AV nodal reentry is usually benign, self-limiting, and easily terminated by a vagal maneuver. However, the arrhythmia may recur frequently, may cause symptoms, and may be refractory to medical therapy. When drug therapy fails to control the arrhythmia, other approaches, such as radiofrequency ablation of one of the two pathways in the AV node, must be considered.

THE WOLFF-PARKINSON-WHITE SYNDROME

Different types of accessory pathways can be present between atrium, AV node, and ventricle.[3] These pathways lead to earlier activation of the ventricle following a supraventricular impulse than during conduction over the AV node (so-called pre-excitation). The most common type of pre-excitation, the Wolff-Parkinson-White (WPW) syndrome, is caused by a direct connection between atrium and ventricle. Such a pathway may be located anywhere atrial and ventricular myocardial tissues are adjacent to each other. Left free wall pathways account for approximately 55 percent of the locations; right free wall, 9 percent; posteroseptal, 33 percent; and anteroseptal, 3 percent.[3]

MECHANISM OF PRE-EXCITATION

Figure 4–4 illustrates the factors that play a role in the electrocardiographic expression of pre-excitation in the presence of a direct connection between

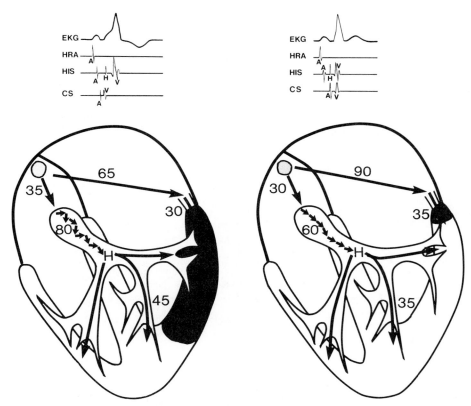

Figure 4–4. A representation of factors determining the degree of ventricular pre-excitation in a patient with Wolff-Parkinson-White syndrome during sinus rhythm. The corresponding ECG and intracavitary recordings from the high right atrium (HRA), His bundle region (HIS), and coronary sinus (CS) are shown in the upper part of the figure. In the heart on the left, AV conduction time from the sinus node over the normal AV nodal–His pathway is 160 msec. The time required to travel from the sinus node to the atrial insertion of the accessory pathway is 65 msec, and the left-sided accessory pathway conduction time is 30 msec (total of 95 msec). Because of the shorter conduction time over the accessory pathway an important part of the ventricle is pre-excited, resulting in a short PR interval, a distinct delta wave, and a widened QRS complex. In the heart to the right, there are a longer conduction time from the sinus node to the atrial insertion of the accessory pathway, a longer conduction time over the accessory pathway itself, and a shorter conduction time over the AV node. Thus, the impulse arrives in the ventricles simultaneously via the AV node and the accessory pathway, producing a normal PR interval and a narrow QRS complex.

atrium and ventricle. As shown in the drawing on the left, a short PR, broad QRS, and a delta wave are present when there is a major contribution (black area in Figure 4–4) to ventricular activation by AV conduction over the accessory pathway. On the right of Figure 4–4, the contribution to ventricular activation over the accessory pathway is minor. This is because the conduction times of the sinus impulse over the AV node and over the accessory pathway to the ventricle are about the same. As shown in Figure 4–5, these differences result in markedly different ECGs. The ECG on the left (Fig. 4–5*A*) clearly shows pre-excitation (overt pre-excitation). This is, however, very difficult to diagnose in the ECG on the right (so-called inapparent or latent pre-excitation). Accessory AV connections do not always conduct in both directions (from atrium to ventricle and ventricle to atrium) but may conduct in one direction only, either anterograde or retrograde. When conduction over the accessory pathway is possible only in the retrograde direction, the term "concealed" accessory AV pathway is used.

CIRCUS MOVEMENT TACHYCARDIA

Normally, supraventricular impulses are conducted to the ventricles only by way of the AV node, resulting in sufficient delay to allow for maximal atrial contribution to ventricular filling. An accessory AV pathway not only short-circuits (pre-excitation) this normal delay in AV conduction, but also creates a pathway for a reentry circuit (so-called circus movement tachycardia).

Circus movement tachycardia may result in narrow or broad QRS tachycardia; both forms are listed below. The narrow QRS circus movement tachycardia is discussed in this chapter. The broad QRS (antidromic) circus movement tachycardia is more extensively discussed in Chapter 3.

PATHWAYS OF CIRCUS MOVEMENT TACHYCARDIA

1. Orthodromic Circus Movement Tachycardia With a Rapidly Conducting Accessory Pathway. AV conduction is over the AV node and VA conduction is over an accessory pathway. The QRS may be narrow or, if there is aberrant ventricular conduction, a typical bundle branch block pattern may be present.

2. Orthodromic Circus Movement Tachycardia With a Slowly Conducting Accessory Pathway. AV conduction is over the AV node, and VA conduction is over an accessory pathway. As with the rapidly conducting accessory pathway, the QRS may be narrow or, if there is aberrant ventricular conduction, a typical bundle branch block pattern may be present.

3. Antidromic Circus Movement Tachycardia, Type 1. AV conduction is over the accessory pathway and VA conduction over the bundle of His and the AV node. This sequence produces a broad QRS tachycardia that is identical in morphology to ventricular tachycardia.

4. Antidromic Circus Movement Tachycardia, Type 2. AV conduction is over one accessory pathway and VA conduction over another accessory pathway. This sequence results in a broad QRS tachycardia that is identical in morphology to ventricular tachycardia.

A

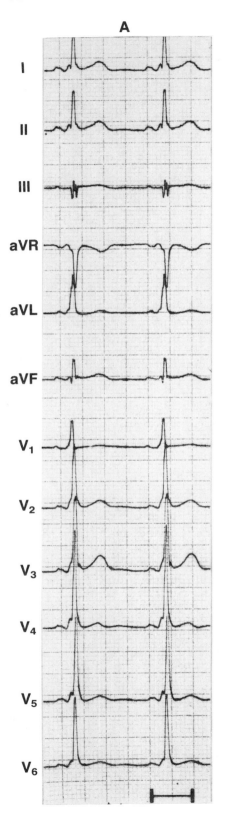

B

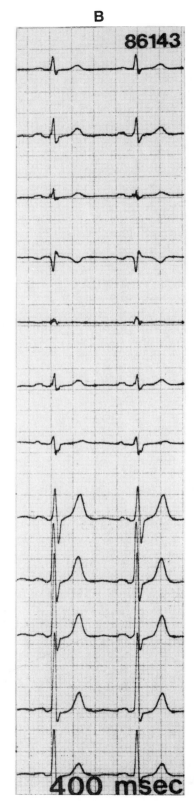

Figure 4–5. Electrocardiographic examples of the two diagrams shown in Figure 4–4. *Panels A* and *B* correspond to the left and right panels, respectively, of Figure 4–4. Note the prominent delta wave in *panel A*, indicating that a much larger area of the ventricle is pre-excited than is shown in *panel B*.

ORTHODROMIC CIRCUS MOVEMENT TACHYCARDIA WITH A RAPIDLY CONDUCTING ACCESSORY PATHWAY

INITIATION AND PERPETUATION

Orthodromic circus movement tachycardia with a rapidly conducting accessory pathway is the most common type of circus movement tachycardia and produces a typical ECG pattern. The tachycardia is initiated by either a PAC or a PVC. Figure 4–6 schematically shows how an orthodromic circus movement tachycardia can be initiated by an atrial or ventricular premature beat.

During orthodromic circus movement tachycardia, activation of the ventricles occurs via the AV node and bundle of His, and therefore the QRS is narrow unless bundle branch block is present. Activation of the atria occurs retrogradely via the accessory pathway, and thus the polarity of the P wave is determined by the location of the atrial insertion of the accessory pathway. Activation of ventricle and activation of atrium follow sequentially so that the P waves are separated from the QRS complexes. Retrograde conduction to the atria occurs rapidly via the accessory pathway, causing the P wave to be closer to the preceding QRS than to the one that follows (RP < PR).

ECG RECOGNITION

- Regular rhythm
- Paroxysmal tachycardia
- QRS less than 0.12 sec, unless bundle branch block is present
- Aberrant ventricular conduction occurs often.
- During narrow QRS circus movement tachycardia, P waves are always separate from the QRS.
- RP less than PR
- P wave axis depends on the location of the accessory pathway. If reentry into the atria is via a left lateral accessory pathway, the P wave is negative in lead I. If the pathway is posteroseptal, the P waves are negative in leads II, III, and aVF.
- QRS alternans is often present (Fig. 4–7), in contrast to AV nodal re-entrant tachycardia, where it is a rare finding after the first 5 seconds of the tachycardia.

It is important to record a 12-lead ECG during the tachycardia because P waves may be clearly visible in one lead but not in another. The same holds true for the phenomenon of electrical alternans.

In the supraventricular tachycardia seen in Figure 4–8A, careful comparison of the ST segments of the tachycardia with those of the sinus rhythm (Fig. 4–8B) reveals a negative P wave separate from the QRS in leads II, III, and aVF, and a positive P wave in leads aVR, aVL, and V_1. QRS alternans is not present in this tracing.

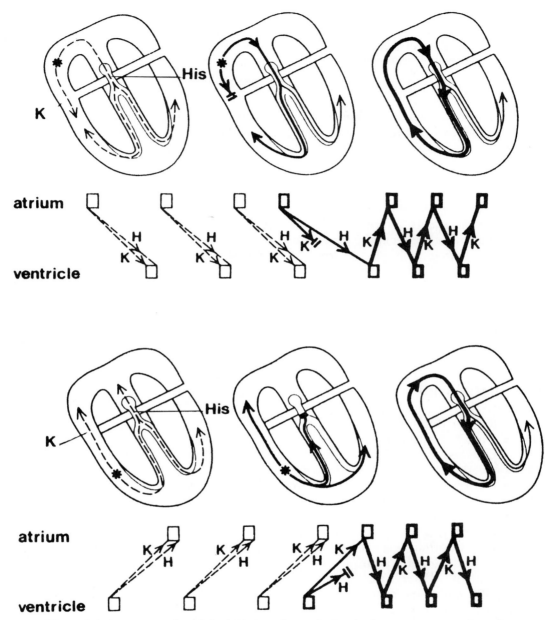

Figure 4–6. A representation of the initiation of an orthodromic circus movement tachycardia (CMT) incorporating an accessory pathway. *(Top)* Initiation by a PAC. Because the refractory period of the accessory pathway (K) is longer than that of the AV nodal–His axis (H), a critically timed PAC is blocked in the accessory pathway (fourth event in the scheme). Following activation of the ventricle over the AV nodal–His pathway, the impulse is conducted back to the atrium over the accessory pathway in the retrograde direction. The impulse is then conducted again to the ventricles over the AV node, and a CMT is initiated. *(Bottom)* Initiation of CMT by a PVC. A critically timed PVC finds the bundle branch–His–AV nodal pathway refractory; it is conducted retrogradely to the atrium over the accessory pathway. Following atrial activation the impulse returns to the ventricle over the AV nodal–His pathway. Perpetuation of this mechanism results in CMT.

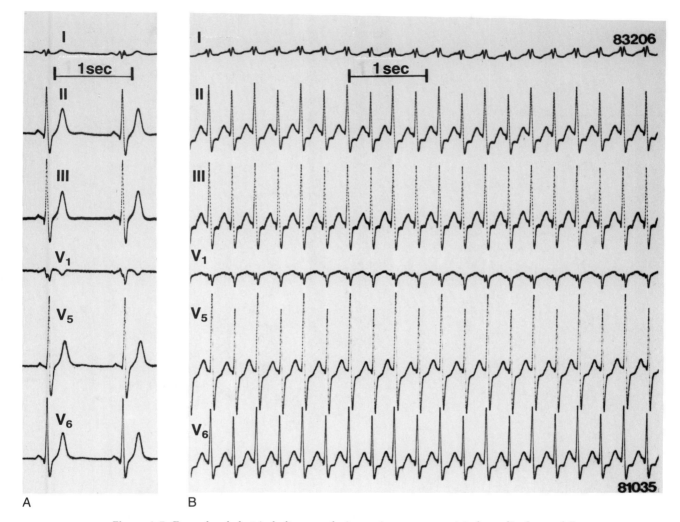

Figure 4–7. Example of electrical alternans during a circus movement tachycardia. In *panel B* several of the leads show alternation in height of successive QRS complexes. Note that the amount of electrical alternans may vary considerably from lead to lead; thus it is necessary to examine each lead carefully for the presence of this phenomenon. *Panel A* is from the same patient during sinus rhythm.

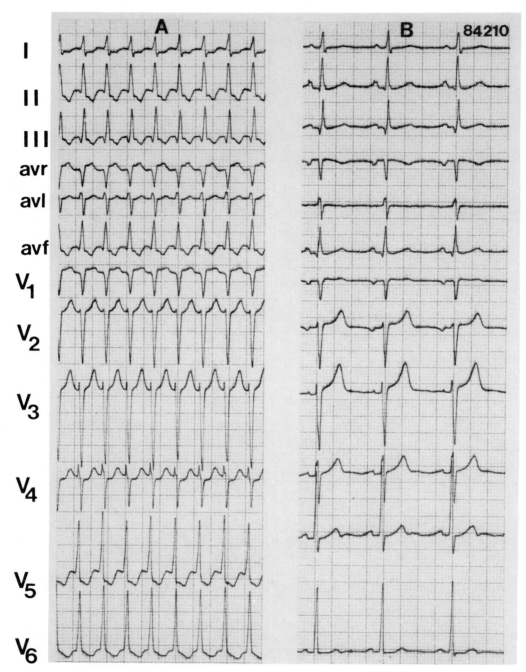

Figure 4–8. An example of a circus movement tachycardia using a concealed accessory pathway. The diagnosis is based on the position of the P waves during the tachycardia *(A)*. Note that when compared with sinus rhythm *(B)*, negative P waves are clearly visible in leads II, III, and aVF following the QRS complex. The P waves during the tachycardia are positive in leads aVR and aVL, indicating a posteroseptal atrial insertion of the accessory pathway.

ORTHODROMIC CIRCUS MOVEMENT TACHYCARDIA WITH A SLOWLY CONDUCTING ACCESSORY PATHWAY; PERSISTENT ("INCESSANT") CIRCUS MOVEMENT TACHYCARDIA

"Incessant" circus movement tachycardia is an arrhythmia that is sustained by a reentry circuit using the AV node in the anterograde direction and a slowly conducting accessory pathway in the retrograde direction. It is important to recognize this relatively rare condition because it frequently does not respond to drugs and may, because of its persistent nature, lead to a dilated cardiomyopathy with congestive heart failure. The arrhythmia can be completely and permanently cured by surgical or electrical ablation of the accessory pathway.

ANATOMICAL SUBSTRATE

The accessory pathway conducts the impulse only from ventricle to atrium (concealed accessory pathway) and is usually located posteroseptally with its atrial insertion close to the ostium of the coronary sinus, producing a typical ECG pattern.

MECHANISM

Orthodromic circus movement tachycardia with a slowly conducting accessory pathway is of a persistent nature (also labeled "incessant" or "permanent") (i.e., the patient is in the tachycardia most of the day).

Impulse conduction over the slowly conducting accessory pathway can be accelerated by atropine, isoprenaline, and exercise. Carotid sinus massage can terminate the circulating impulse both in the AV node and in the accessory pathway. These properties, which do not apply to rapidly conducting accessory pathways, suggest that the slowly conducting accessory pathway behaves like AV nodal tissue.

A premature atrial complex (PAC) is not necessary to begin this tachycardia; it can start spontaneously following a sinus beat (Fig. 4–9). The impulse passes in an anterograde direction down the AV node to activate the ventricles and then returns to the atria via the slowly conducting accessory pathway.

ECG RECOGNITION

- Regular rhythm
- Persistent in nature
- QRS less than 0.12 sec, unless bundle branch block is present
- P waves always separate from the QRS
- RP greater than PR
- P waves negative in leads II, III, aVF, and V_3 to V_6

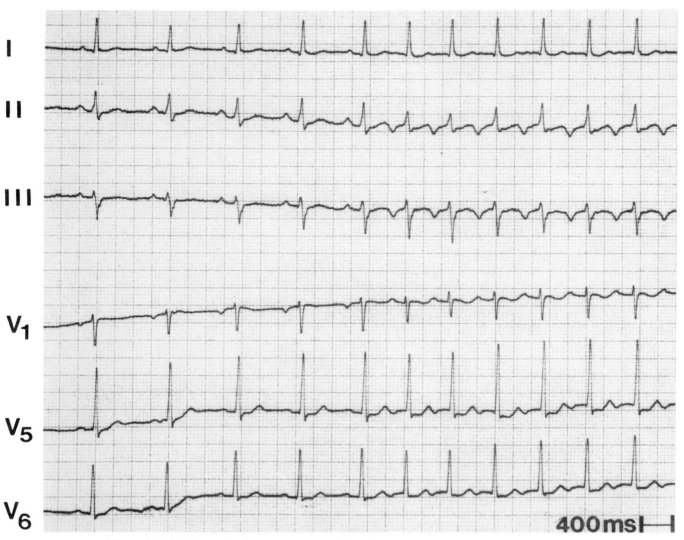

Figure 4–9. Initiation of a circus movement tachycardia using a slowly conducting concealed accessory pathway. Note that an increase in sinus rate is sufficient to initiate the tachycardia. During tachycardia the P waves are negative in leads II, III, V_5, and V_6, and the RP interval is longer than the PR interval.

The tachycardias shown in Figures 4–10 and 4–11 are examples of circus movement tachycardia using a slowly conducting concealed accessory pathway in the retrograde direction. The diagnosis is made because of the (1) incessant nature of the tachycardia, (2) polarity of the P waves during the tachycardia, and (3) long RP interval.

The negative P waves in the inferior leads indicate that activation of the atria is initiated low in the atrium close to the mouth of the coronary sinus. Since retrograde conduction over the accessory pathway is slow, the P wave is closer to the QRS that follows than to the preceding one (RP greater than PR). Table 4–2 summarizes the ECG features of narrow QRS tachycardia.

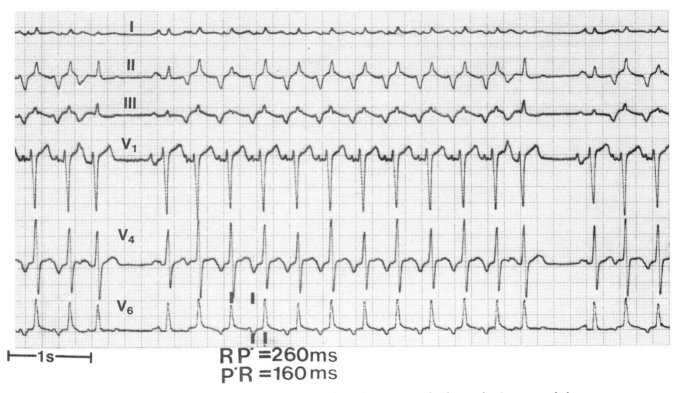

RP´=260ms
P´R =160ms

Figure 4–10. Incessant circus movement tachycardia using a slowly conducting concealed accessory pathway for retrograde conduction. The diagnosis is made because the patient is in tachycardia most of the time with an RP interval greater than PR. The tachycardia is temporarily terminated by an atrial premature beat, which is conducted to the ventricle. There is a pause due to retrograde block in the accessory pathway. Then the sinus node escapes for one beat and the circus movement tachycardia begins again.

Table 4–2. **Summary of the ECG Features of Narrow QRS Tachycardias**

ECG Signs	AVNRT	CMT (Incorporating Accessory Pathway)	Atrial Tachycardia
AV block (spontaneous or by CSM)	Usually not but 2:1 is possible	Rules out CMT	If present, atrial rate >250 = atrial flutter; atrial rate <250 = atrial tachycardia
Electrical alternans	Rare	Common (especially at high rates)	Rare
P wave location	Hidden in the QRS or distorting the distal (common) or proximal (uncommon) portion of the QRS	Present between the R waves; usually (fast AP) RP <PR, uncommon form (slow AP) RP >PR	Present between R waves; PR duration varies with site of origin and AV nodal conduction time
P polarity	Always negative in leads II, III, and aVF	Varies according to location of the accessory pathway	Varies with the location of the atrial focus, but in digitalis toxicity, often almost identical to sinus P wave (Chapter 8)
Aberrancy	Rare	Common	Rare

AP—accessory pathway; AVNRT—AV nodal reentry tachycardia; CSM—carotid sinus massage; CMT—circus movement tachycardia.

SYSTEMATIC APPROACH TO THE PATIENT WITH NARROW QRS TACHYCARDIA

A systematic approach permits correct identification of the site of origin or pathway of the narrow QRS tachycardia in 85 percent of patients.[5] Such a four-step approach during tachycardia is summarized in Table 4–3 and involves an evaluation of (1) spontaneous AV block or that induced by carotid sinus massage, (2) QRS alternans, (3) P wave location, and (4) P wave polarity.

1. IS THERE AV BLOCK?

AV block rules out circus movement tachycardia. When AV block is present, the atrial rate helps to make the differential diagnosis; rates over 250 beats per minute suggest atrial flutter, and rates lower than that suggest atrial tachycardia. AV nodal reentry with 2:1 block below the AV node is rare but possible.

2. IS THERE QRS ALTERNANS?

QRS alternans during narrow QRS tachycardia has been demonstrated to have a high degree of specificity for orthodromic circus movement tachycardia and is therefore helpful in differentiating this type of tachycardia from other types.[5, 6]

Table 4–3. **Steps in the Diagnosis of a Regular Narrow QRS in Tachycardia**

Question	Answer	Diagnosis
If second-degree AV block (spontaneous or after CSM) **what is the atrial rate?**	250/min or more	Atrial flutter
	<250/min	Arial tachycardia AVNRT with 2:1 block (rare)
Is there QRS alternation?	No	Inconclusive
	Yes	CMT
Where is the P wave located?	PR > RP	CMT with fast AP
	P in R	AVNRT
	PR < RP	Atrial tachycardia or CMT with slow AP
What is the frontal plane axis?	Inferior-superior	Atrial tachycardia or CMT with slow or fast (septal) AP
	Other	Atrial tachycardia or CMT with fast AP (right or left)
What is the horizontal plane axis?	Right to left	Right atrial tachycardia or CMT with fast AP (right)
	Left to right	CMT (fast left AP) or left atrial tachycardia

AP—accessory pathway; AVNRT—AV nodal reentry tachycardia; CMT—circus movement tachycardia; CSM—carotid sinus massage.

QRS alternans, which is found particularly at high heart rates (above 200 per minute), occurs in approximately 30 percent of circus movement tachycardias and is rare in AV nodal reentry. However, the finding of QRS alternans can only be used as a clue to the diagnosis of circus movement tachycardia if the alternans is still present after the first 5 seconds of the tachycardia. This is because changes in height and configuration of the QRS are common in the first seconds after the start of any type of supraventricular tachycardia.

3. WHERE IS THE P WAVE RELATIVE TO THE QRS?

P Wave Within the QRS. If the P wave is within or distorting the beginning or end of the QRS, the arrhythmia can be diagnosed as AV nodal reentry tachycardia.

P Wave Separate From the QRS and RP<PR. If the P wave is separate from the QRS and the RP is less than the PR, the mechanism is circus movement tachycardia (using a fast accessory pathway).

P Wave Separate From QRS and RP>PR. If the P wave is separate from the QRS and the RP is greater than the PR, the mechanism may be one of three possibilities: (1) circus movement tachycardia using a slowly conducting accessory pathway, (2) the uncommon form of AV nodal reentry tachycardia, or (3) atrial tachycardia, in which case the length of the PR interval is determined by the site of atrial impulse formation and time taken for AV nodal transmission.

Figure 4–11 illustrates two cases of supraventricular tachycardia. In Figure 4–11A, AV nodal reentry is present; note that the P wave is distorting the end of the QRS during the tachycardia, looking like an r' wave in lead V₁ and an S wave in leads II, III, and aVF. Figure 4–11B shows orthodromic circus movement tachycardia. The P waves are clearly separate from the QRS and can be seen distorting the ST segment.

4. WHAT IS THE POLARITY (AXIS) OF THE P WAVE?

Vertical (Frontal Plane). A frontal plane P axis that is vertical (positive P waves in leads II, III, and aVF) rules out both AV nodal reentry tachycardia and circus movement tachycardia and indicates atrial tachycardia. (See also Chapter 8 for atrial tachycardia due to digitalis toxicity.)

Inferior/Superior (Frontal Plane). A frontal plane P wave axis that is inferior to superior (negative P waves in leads II, III, aVF) could be the result of either AV nodal reentry tachycardia or circus movement tachycardia using a posteroseptal accessory pathway.

Right to Left (Horizontal Plane). In the horizontal plane, a right-to-left P wave axis (positive P wave in leads I and aVL) rules out AV nodal reentry; such an axis can be found in either right atrial tachycardia or circus movement tachycardia using a right-sided accessory pathway.

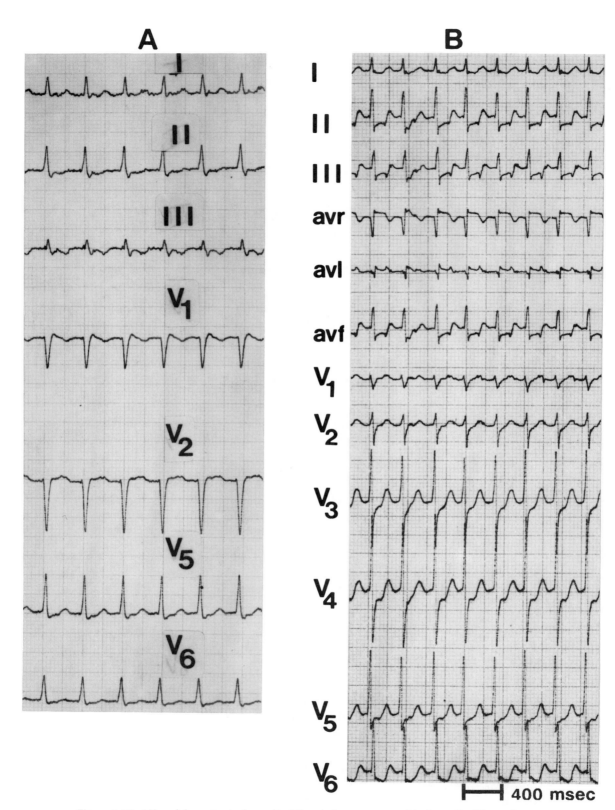

Figure 4–11. AV nodal reentry tachycardia *(A)* and circus movement tachycardia *(B)* are shown for comparison. *(A)* Note that during AV nodal reentry tachycardia the P wave is distorting the end of the QRS (S in leads II and III and r' in lead V_1). *(B)* In circus movement tachycardia the P waves are clearly separate from the QRS and can easily be seen in leads II, III, aVL, and aVF.

Left to Right (Horizontal Plane). A left-to-right axis (negative P wave in leads I and aVL) could be circus movement tachycardia using a left-sided accessory pathway or left atrial tachycardia.

ABERRANT VENTRICULAR CONDUCTION, A HELPFUL CLUE

Ventricular aberration is more common in circus movement tachycardia than it is in AV nodal reentry tachycardia. The reason is explained in Figure 4–12. When episodes of aberrant and nonaberrant conduction are present in the same patient during tachycardia, it is very important to compare the heart rates under both circumstances. If aberration (bundle branch block) is on the same side as the accessory pathway, the rate is slower during aberrant ventricular conduction than it is without aberration because of the larger circuit that the impulse travels due to the blocked bundle branch (Fig. 4–13). Such a finding not only is diagnostic of circus movement tachycardia but also identifies the accessory pathway as inserting in the free wall of either the right or the left ventricle. For example, a slowing of the rate during

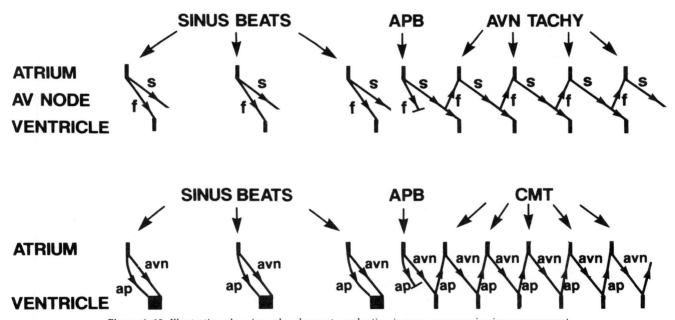

Figure 4–12. Illustration showing why aberrant conduction is more common in circus movement tachycardia than in AV nodal reentry tachycardia. *(Top)* A ladder diagram of initiation of the common type of AV nodal reentry tachycardia (AVNRT) by an APB. Following the APB, the change from conduction over the fast to the slow AV nodal pathway results in a relatively long coupling interval at the ventricular level between the conducted APB and the preceding QRS, making phase 3 block in the bundle branch unlikely. *(Bottom)* Initiation of a circus movement tachycardia (CMT) by an APB. Initiation occurs because the APB is blocked in the accessory pathway in the anterograde direction. Conduction over the AV node results in a relatively short coupling interval of the conducted APB to the preceding QRS complex favoring the occurrence of phase 3 block in the bundle branch. Persistence of aberrant conduction during tachycardia is frequently based on retrograde invasion into the bundle branch (see Chapter 3).

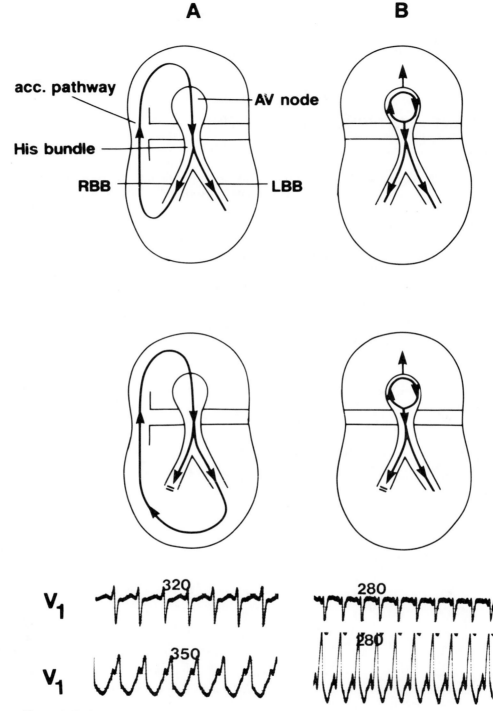

Figure 4–13. A representation of the increase in the length of the reentry circuit when bundle branch block develops during circus movement tachycardia using an accessory (acc.) pathway that is on the same side as the bundle branch block. In *A* there is a right-sided accessory pathway. In *B* the tachycardia circuit is confined to the AV node. When right bundle branch block develops in the patient with a right-sided accessory pathway, the circuit becomes longer and the tachycardia rate slows (compare V_1 before and after right bundle branch block on the left). In contrast (shown in *B*), nothing happens with the tachycardia rate when bundle branch block develops during AV nodal reentrant tachycardia. (Measurements are in msec.)

circus movement tachycardia because of right bundle branch block (Fig. 4–14) indicates a right free wall accessory pathway; a slowing because of left bundle branch block (Fig. 4–15) indicates a left free wall accessory pathway. Of course, if bundle branch block is on one side and the accessory pathway on the other, there will be no slowing during aberration.

SYSTEMATIC APPROACH TO TREATMENT IN SUPRAVENTRICULAR TACHYCARDIA

1. Record a 12-lead ECG.
2. Physical examination: if the ECG does not allow proper diagnosis of the site of origin of the narrow QRS tachycardia because P waves cannot be identified, evaluate the jugular pulse; the "frog sign" indicates either AV nodal reentry tachycardia or circus movement tachycardia. Flutter waves in the jugular pulse indicate atrial flutter.

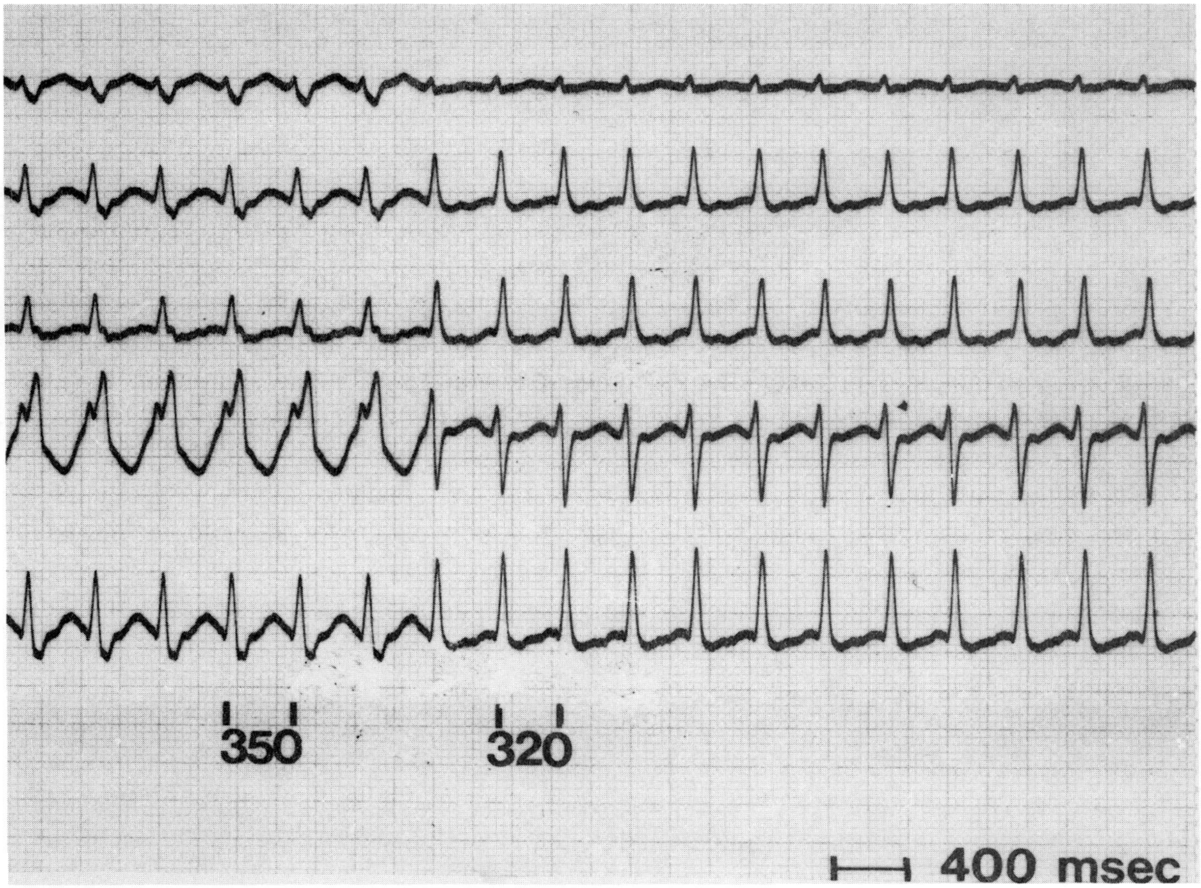

Figure 4–14. Circus movement tachycardia with right bundle branch block aberration. Note that the rate is slower during the aberration than during the tachycardia without aberration. This indicates the presence of a right-sided accessory pathway. (Measurements are in msec.)

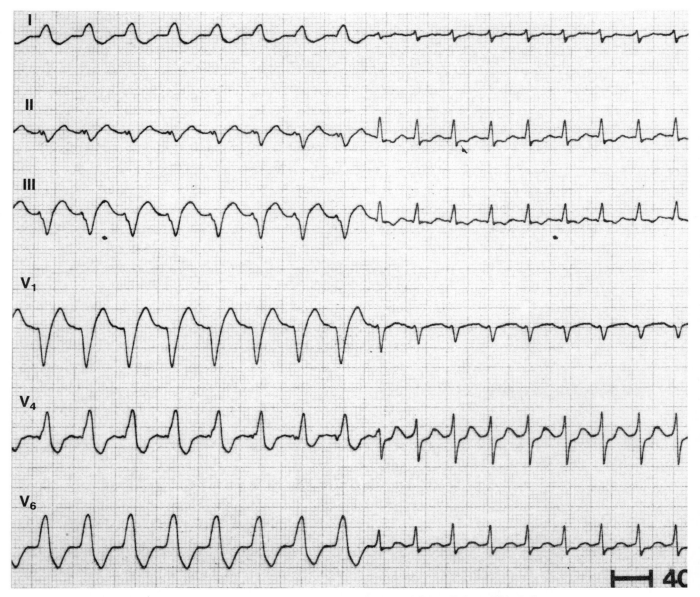

Figure 4–15. Circus movement tachycardia with and without left bundle branch block aberration. Note that the rate of the tachycardia is slower during left bundle branch block, indicating the presence of a left-sided accessory pathway.

3. Apply a vagal maneuver; if unsuccessful:

4. Inject 6 mg of adenosine over 1 to 2 sec. If supraventricular tachycardia is not terminated in 1 to 2 minutes, inject 12 mg of adenosine as a rapid IV bolus; this dose may be repeated once. Adenosine has a half-life of less than 1.5 seconds so that the adverse reactions (facial flushing, dyspnea) last only a short time.[7] If adenosine is not available:

5. Inject 10 mg of verapamil IV over a 3-minute period. In case of previous use of a beta blocking drug or hypotension, reduce the dose of verapamil to 5 mg (inject over a 5-minute period).

6. When the tachycardia is not terminated, inject procainamide IV (10 mg/kg body weight) over a 5-minute period.

7. Cardiovert if the tachycardia persists and the patient is deteriorating hemodynamically.

8. Once the tachycardia has been terminated, record the 12-lead ECG in sinus rhythm so that P waves during the tachycardia can more easily be located; this is best done by comparing the QRS and ST-T segments during tachycardia with those of the sinus rhythm.

PERSISTENT ("INCESSANT") ATRIAL TACHYCARDIA

"Incessant" atrial tachycardia is an arrhythmia of unknown mechanism arising in the atrium and eventually leading to congestive cardiomyopathy because of its persistent nature. Recognition is very important because surgical removal of the area of abnormal impulse formation results in cure of the arrhythmia and in complete regression of congestive heart failure.

ECG RECOGNITION

Rhythm. Regular.

P Waves. In front of the QRS; configuration and polarity depend upon the site of origin in the atrium.

AV Conduction. May vary (1:1, 2:1, Wenckebach conduction).

Carotid Sinus Massage. Increases AV block, facilitating recognition of the atrial origin of the arrhythmia.

VAGAL STIMULATION

The vagal nerve is part of the parasympathetic nervous system, the mediator of which is acetylcholine. Both the sinus and AV nodes are richly supplied with autonomic nerves and are especially sensitive to acetylcholine. Vagal maneuvers cause the parasympathetic nerves to release acetylcholine, which blocks or delays conduction in the AV node.

When a vagal maneuver causes complete AV block, it terminates circus movement tachycardia or AV nodal reentry tachycardia. If the tachycardia circuit does not involve the AV node (atrial tachycardia or atrial flutter), the vagal maneuver exposes the site of origin of the arrhythmia in case of the creation of AV block.

TYPES OF VAGAL MANEUVERS

Some of the vagal maneuvers are:

1. Carotid sinus massage
2. Gagging (by placing the finger in the throat)
3. Valsalva maneuver (blowing against a closed glottis; squatting)
4. Trendelenburg position
5. The dive reflex (facial immersion in cold water)
6. Coughing

Note. Eyeball pressure is *not* an acceptable vagal maneuver; it is unpleasant for the patient, is rarely effective, and may cause retinal detachment.

CAROTID SINUS MASSAGE

The carotid sinus (Fig. 4–16) is located at the bifurcation of the carotid artery just below the angle of the jaw. In the hands of the informed health professional, carotid sinus stimulation is an excellent diagnostic and therapeutic vagotonic maneuver. Its purpose is to create an elevation of blood pressure in the carotid sinus so that acetylcholine is released, causing slowing or block of AV conduction, which will terminate AV nodal reentry tachycardia and circus movement tachycardia and expose the atrial activity of atrial flutter and atrial fibrillation.

HOW TO PERFORM CAROTID SINUS MASSAGE

PALPATE AND AUSCULTATE THE CAROTID ARTERIES

1. Before commencing carotid sinus massage, try to exclude stenosis of one of the carotid arteries by palpation and by listening for carotid bruits; if possible, take a history that will reveal any transient ischemic attacks. Such a finding is a contraindication for carotid sinus massage.
2. Monitor the effect of carotid sinus massage on the ECG; if an ECG is not available, listen to the heart with the stethoscope as you massage the carotid sinus.

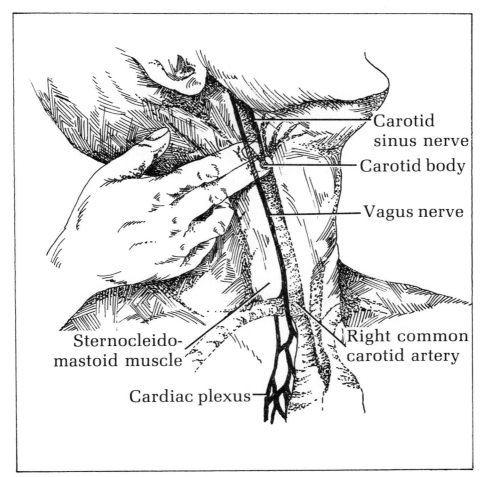

Figure 4–16. Location of the carotid body and position of the fingers for carotid sinus massage. (From Conover, M.: Understanding Electrocardiography, 5th ed. St. Louis, 1988, C.V. Mosby.)

PRECAUTIONS

1. Pressure applied for longer than 5 seconds may be dangerous.
2. Beware of performing this maneuver in patients over 65 years of age because long sinus pauses may result (pauses of 3–7 sec have been reported).

CORRECT POSITIONING OF THE PATIENT

1. Place the patient in a horizontal position with the neck extended; this is achieved with either a small pillow or an arm under the patient's shoulders.
2. Turn the patient's head away from the side to be massaged.

CORRECT TECHNIQUE

1. Locate the bifurcation of the carotid artery just below the angle of the jaw. Figure 4–16 shows an approach from behind the patient.
2. Massage one side at a time.
3. Begin with only slight pressure in the event of a hypersensitive patient. Thereafter, apply firm pressure with a massaging action for no more than 5 seconds. Firm pressure is achieved by pressing the carotid sinus against the lateral processes of the vertebrae. Such a maneuver will cause pain, and the patient should be warned of this and told that it will last for only a few seconds.

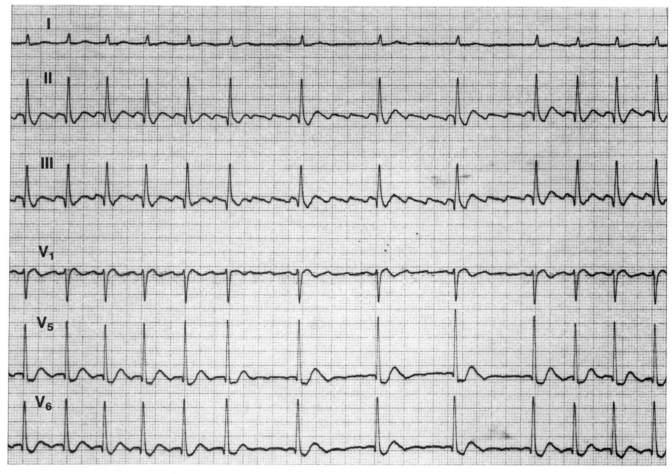

Figure 4–17. Carotid sinus massage (CSM) slows conduction through the AV node, revealing an underlying atrial flutter. Six ECG leads were recorded simultaneously.

EFFECT OF CAROTID SINUS MASSAGE ON SUPRAVENTRICULAR TACHYCARDIA

Carotid sinus massage causes:

1. Either temporary slowing of the ventricular rate due to AV block (Fig. 4–17) or it has no effect on atrial flutter, atrial fibrillation, and the incessant form of atrial tachycardia; it may also convert atrial flutter to atrial fibrillation.
2. Gradual and temporary slowing of the heart rate during sinus tachycardia (Fig. 4–18).

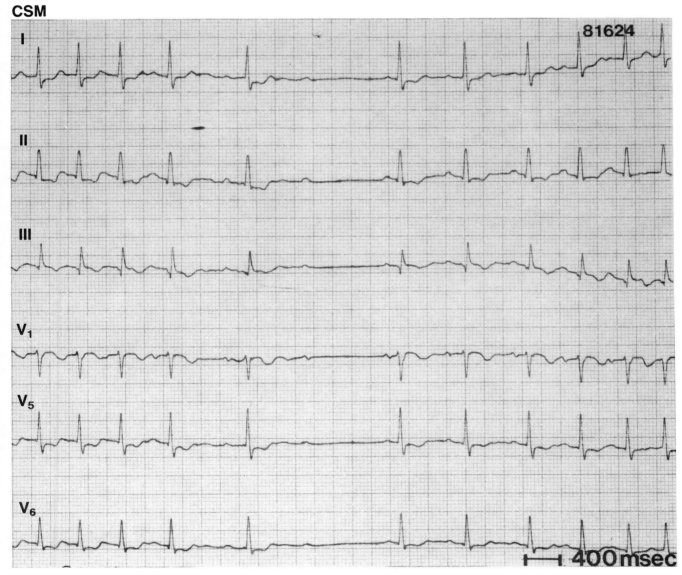

Figure 4–18. Carotid sinus massage (CSM) causes gradual slowing of the rate of the sinus node during sinus tachycardia.

CSM

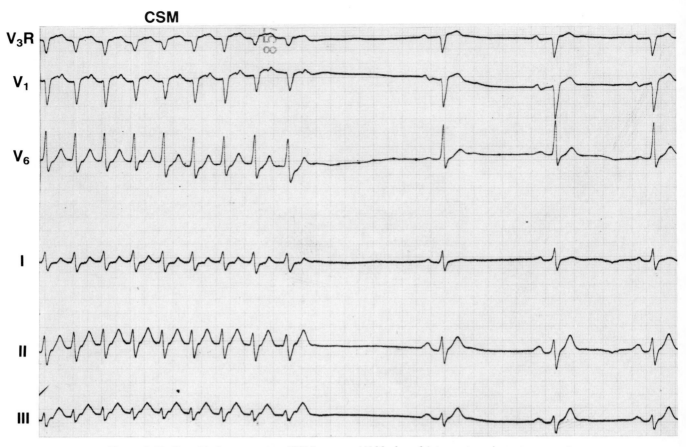

Figure 4–19. Carotid sinus massage (CSM) causes AV block and interrupts a circus movement tachycardia, using a concealed accessory pathway for VA conduction.

3. Abrupt cessation of AV nodal reentry tachycardia and circus movement tachycardia (Fig. 4–19) or it may have no effect. Carotid sinus massage terminates these tachycardias because of block in the AV node. These effects are summarized in Table 4–4.

Table 4–4. **Effect of Carotid Sinus Massage on Supraventricular Tachycardia**[2]

Type of SVT	Effect of CSM
Sinus tachycardia	Gradual and temporary slowing in heart rate
Atrial tachycardia	
Paroxysmal	Cessation of tachycardia or no effect
Incessant	Temporary slowing of ventricular rate (AV block) or no effect
Atrial flutter	Temporary slowing of ventricular rate (AV block), conversion into atrial fibrillation, or no effect
Atrial fibrillation	Temporary slowing of ventricular rate (AV block) or no effect
AVNRT	Cessation of tachycardia or no effect
CMT	Cessation of tachycardia or no effect

AVNRT—AV nodal reentry tachycardia; CMT—circus movement tachycardia (using an accessory pathway and the AV node).

Data from Wellens, H.J.J., Brugada, P., and Bar, F.: Diagnosis and treatment of the regular tachycardia with a narrow QRS complex. In Kalbertus, H.E. (ed.): Medical Management of Cardiac Arrhythmias. Edinburgh, 1986, Churchill-Livingstone.

SUMMARY

Narrow QRS tachycardia is faster than 100 beats per minute with a QRS duration of less than 0.12 sec. It may be due to sinus or atrial tachycardia, atrial flutter or fibrillation, AV nodal tachycardia, or orthodromic circus movement tachycardia. The two most common causes of a regular paroxysmal supraventricular tachycardia are AV nodal reentry and orthodromic circus movement using an accessory pathway in the retrograde direction and the AV node in the anterograde direction.

A systematic approach to the differential diagnosis during paroxysmal supraventricular tachycardia involves queries as to the presence or induction (by vagal maneuvers) of AV block; QRS alternans; observations regarding the position and polarity of the P wave; and the response to vagal maneuvers.

A systematic approach to the treatment of paroxysmal supraventricular tachycardia requires a 12-lead ECG, physical examination, and a vagal maneuver. When vagal maneuvers are unsuccessful, adenosine, verapamil, or procainamide is used and then cardioversion is performed, if necessary.

References

1. Harvey, W.P., and Ronan, J.A.: Bedside diagnosis of arrhythmias. Prog. Cardiovasc. Dis. 8:419–431, 1966.
2. Wellens, H.J.J., Brugada, P., and Bar, F.: Diagnosis and treatment of the regular tachycardia with a narrow QRS complex. In Kulbertus, H.E. (ed.): Medical Management of Cardiac Arrhythmias. Edinburgh, 1986, Churchill Livingstone, pp. 121–132.
3. Wellens, H.J.J., Brugada, P., and Penn, O.C.: The management of preexcitation syndromes. J.A.M.A. 257:2325–2333, 1987.
4. Wellens, H.J.J., Atie, J., Penn, O.C., et al.: Diagnosis and treatment of patients with accessory pathways. Cardiol. Clin. 8:503–521, 1990.
5. Bar, F.W., Brugada, P., Dassen, W.R.M., et al.: Differential diagnosis of tachycardia with narrow QRS complex (shorter than 0.12 second). Am. J. Cardiol. 54;555–560, 1984.
6. Green, M., Heddle, B., Dassen, W., et al.: Value of QRS alternation in determining the site of origin of narrow QRS supraventricular tachycardia. Circulation 68:368–373, 1983.
7. Lerman, B.B., and Belardinelli, L.: Cardiac electrophysiology of adenosine. Basic and clinical concepts. Circulation 83:1499–1509, 1991.

CHAPTER

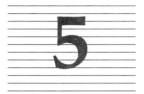

5

Slow Atrial Rhythms

EMERGENCY APPROACH

1. Record a 12-lead ECG.
2. In case of hypotension and other signs of diminished cardiac output, immediately initiate the following supportive measures: Give IV atropine 0.04 mg/kg body weight. If heart rate does not accelerate, temporary pacing is indicated.
3. If hypotension, dizziness, and presyncope are absent, no immediate treatment is required.
4. Evaluate ECG for:
   - Myocardial infarction
   - Mechanism of bradycardia: Note regularity, abrupt pauses, or group beating. P wave regularity indicates a regular sinus or atrial rhythm; abrupt pauses in the sinus rhythm or group beating suggests SA block; abrupt pauses or group beating in the ventricular rhythm suggests AV block.
   - QRS axis and width for coexistent bundle branch block
5. If sinus bradycardia is demonstrated, give no treatment unless hypotension is present (give atropine).
6. In case of SA block or sinus arrest, give no treatment unless hypotension is present or the rhythm is digitalis-induced (stop the drug).
7. If the diagnosis is sick sinus syndrome, treatment will depend upon symptoms (dizziness, presyncope, congestive failure).

SINUS BRADYCARDIA

ECG RECOGNITION

Sinus bradycardia is a regular sinus rhythm with a rate of less than 60 beats per minute. The P waves are uniform in shape, originating from the sinus node. The rhythm is regular unless sinus arrhythmia is also present.

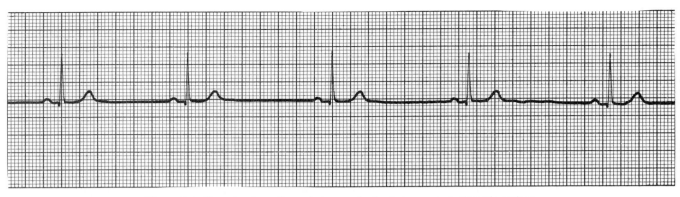

Figure 5–1. Sinus bradycardia and sinus arrhythmia in an asymptomatic patient.

CLINICAL IMPLICATIONS

Sinus bradycardia occurs normally in trained athletes and during sleep, or it may be due to one of a number of causes, among which are the effects of drugs, hypothyroidism, and hypothermia. Figure 5–1 shows an example of sinus bradycardia. Among the common drugs that may cause sinus brady-cardia are digitalis (due to SA block) and beta blocking agents.

In acute myocardial infarction, especially during the first hours following inferior wall myocardial infarction, sinus bradycardia is common (10–40 percent) and is usually the result of increased vagal tone caused by pain and anxiety. Figure 5–2 illustrates a sinus bradycardia during acute inferior wall myocardial infarction.

MANAGEMENT

Treatment of sinus bradycardia depends on whether there is hypotension. If the sinus bradycardia is well tolerated, no treatment is indicated. If it is not tolerated (if there is diaphoresis, lightheadedness, etc.), or when sinus bradycardia is associated with hypotension in the presence of myocardial infarction, intravenous atropine (0.04 mg/kg body weight) is the drug of choice.

In digitalis toxicity, treatment involves discontinuing the drug, bedrest, and continuous monitoring (see Chapter 8). If hypotension is a factor, digitalis antibodies or pacing may be indicated.

SECOND-DEGREE SINOATRIAL BLOCK AND SINUS ARREST

Second-degree sinoatrial (SA) block and sinus arrest are both manifested by dropped P waves. Second-degree SA block is a disorder of conduction (the impulses are generated but not conducted) and may be either type I or type II; sinus arrest is a disorder of automaticity (the impulses are not generated).

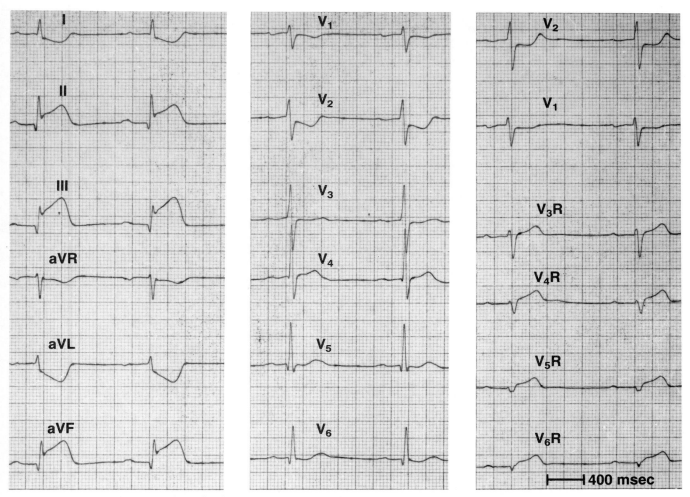

Figure 5–2. Sinus bradycardia in a patient with acute inferior wall myocardial infarction. Note that the elevated ST segment in lead V_4R indicates a proximal occlusion in the right coronary artery. (See also Chapter 1.)

Types I and II second-degree SA block are differentiated from each other because of the pattern of the PP intervals prior to the missing P wave. Direct recordings of the sinus node reveal the mechanisms of SA block and sinus arrest.[1, 2]

CAUSES

There are many known causes for SA block or sinus arrest. They include

> Excessive vagal stimulation
> Carotid hypersensitivity
> Myocardial infarction
> Acute myocarditis
> Hyper- or hypokalemia

Tumor

Inflammation

Drugs, such as beta blocking agents, calcium channel blockers, digitalis, quinidine, acetylcholine, all class IA agents (quinidine, procainamide, disopyramide), class IC agents (flecainide, encainide, lorcainide, propafenone, indecainide), rarely class IB agents, amiodarone, sotalol, and lithium

MANAGEMENT

Management of patients with SA block or sinus arrest depends on the hemodynamic consequences of the rhythm. If the patient is hemodynamically unstable, a pacemaker is indicated.

TYPE I SECOND-DEGREE SINOATRIAL BLOCK

ECG RECOGNITION

In type I SA block (SA Wenckebach) there are shortening PP intervals and pauses that are less than twice the shortest cycle. Figure 5–3 is an example of type I second-degree SA block. The PR intervals are not affected by this condition unless there is an additional AV nodal conduction problem.

Type I SA block with 2:1 exit block must be differentiated from bigeminal nonconducted PACs by carefully examining the shape of the T waves for hidden ectopic P waves.

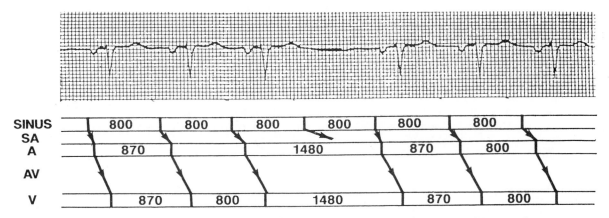

Figure 5–3. SA Wenckebach. Note the group beating, shortening of successive PP intervals, and pauses that are less than twice the shortest cycle. The ladder diagram illustrates the mechanism. Note that the sinus node is firing at regular intervals (800 msec), but that because of Wenckebach conduction from the sinus node to the atrial tissue, with the largest increment between the first and second beats of the group, the PP intervals shorten. The pause represents a sinus beat that was not conducted to the atria.

MECHANISM

The mechanism of SA Wenckebach is easily explained because of the type of tissue involved. Sinus nodal cells are similar to AV nodal cells, and conduction velocity through this tissue is normally slow. Thus, conduction defects between the sinus node and atrial muscle tissue behave very much the same as do conduction problems originating in the AV node, but without the PR prolongation or progressive PR lengthening. For example, first-degree SA block would exist when the time between the firing of the sinus node and activation of the atria is abnormally long. Although laboratory studies have defined what the normal SA conduction should be, the discharge of the SA node is not seen on the surface ECG. However, it is possible to recognize second-degree SA block on the surface ECG because P waves are intermittently missing.

The Wenckebach conduction phenomenon can be found anywhere there are slow response action potentials, normally in the sinus node and the AV node and abnormally in damaged (for example, ischemic) tissue. Wenckebach conduction consists of a cyclic lengthening of conduction time until conduction finally does not occur (a "dropped" beat) and the cycle begins again.

TYPE II SECOND-DEGREE SINOATRIAL BLOCK

ECG RECOGNITION

In type II SA block there is a regular sinus rhythm that is interrupted by a pause that is a multiple of the rate of the sinus rhythm. Figure 5–4 is an example of type II second-degree SA block.

Type II SA block is differentiated from nonconducted PACs by making sure that all P waves have normal sinus configuration and none are premature. The T wave preceding the pause should be examined for nonconducted PACs before a diagnosis of SA block is made.

MECHANISM

In type II SA block the sinus node is firing on time but SA conduction fails intermittently for one or two beats.

COMPLETE SINOATRIAL BLOCK

In complete SA block, conduction between the sinus node and atrial tissue fails completely; that is, there are no sinus P waves, although an atrial escape rhythm may occur. In case of digitalis toxicity, complete SA block may be masked by coexisting impulse formation in the atria and/or AV junction (atrial tachycardia and/or junctional tachycardia). The mechanism and arrhythmias of digitalis toxicity are discussed in detail in Chapter 8.

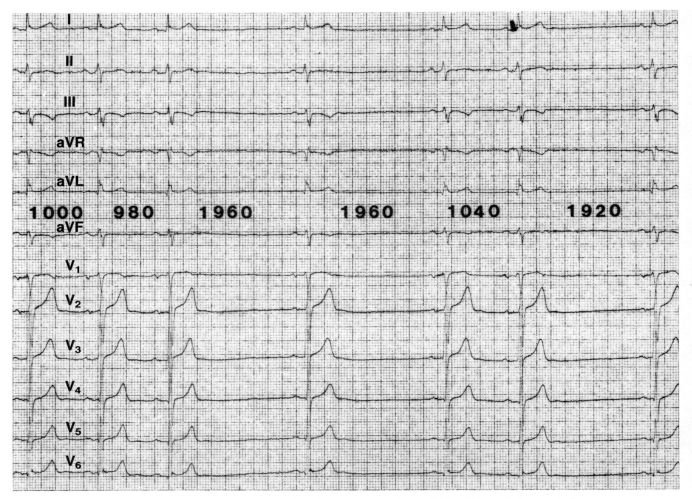

Figure 5–4. Type II SA block. Note that the pause is an exact multiple of the uninterrupted PP interval. Presumably a sinus discharge occurred on time but was not conducted to the surrounding atrial tissue, resulting in an absent P wave. The measurements are in milliseconds.

SINUS ARREST

In sinus arrest, sinus impulses are not formed, resulting in a junctional escape rhythm as seen in Figure 5–5, or resulting in pauses during regular sinus rhythm that are not numerically related to the basic cycle length.

The distinction between SA exit block and sinus arrest is not possible to determine with certainty on the surface ECG (Fig. 5–5). Additionally, many of the conditions that produce sinus arrest are also capable of lengthening the sinus cycle and influencing SA conduction, such as the intense vagal tone that results from a hypersensitive carotid sinus.

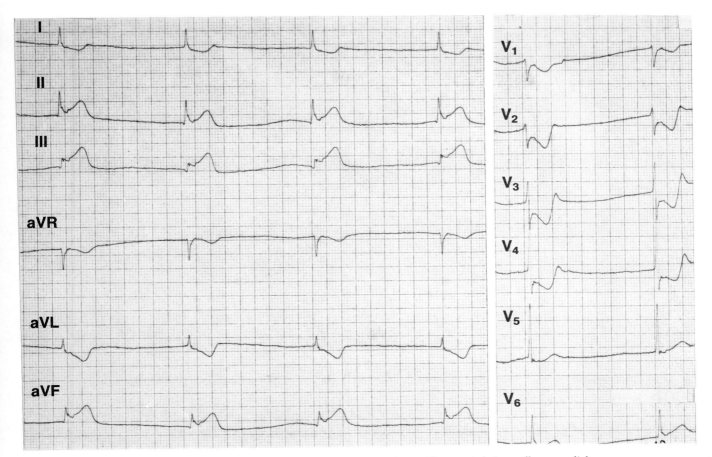

Figure 5–5. Complete SA block or sinus arrest in a patient with acute inferior wall myocardial infarction. There is a junctional escape rhythm with retrograde P waves at the end of the QRS complex.

SICK SINUS SYNDROME

The term "sick sinus syndrome" (SSS)[3] is used when a patient presents with dizziness or lightheadedness secondary to sinus nodal dysfunction and failure of adequate escape pacemakers. The condition may involve a combination of SA nodal, atrial, and AV junctional disease.

ECG RECOGNITION

SSS is diagnosed when cerebral perfusion is inadequate because of any of the following arrhythmias:

1. Marked or inappropriate sinus bradycardia. Sinus bradycardia is marked when it is persistent at less than 40 beats per minute and inappropriate when the heart rate fails to accelerate during exercise or fever.

2. Marked or inappropriate sinus arrhythmia. A slowing to a rate of less than 40 beats per minute that produces symptoms or pauses of more than 2 sec is rare in normal individuals, with the exception of endurance athletes, and suggests sinus node dysfunction.
3. Sinus arrest or SA block
4. Slow atrial rhythm with an unreliable junctional escape rhythm
5. Bradycardia-tachycardia syndrome. In this arrhythmia, bradycardia alternates with tachycardia. The tachycardia phase of this arrhythmia is frequently paroxysmal atrial fibrillation but may be any other type of supraventricular tachycardia. Following cessation of the tachycardia there is an excessively long pause before an escape rhythm starts.

CLINICAL IMPLICATIONS

SSS is caused by abnormalities in SA automaticity and SA conduction and failure of adequate escape mechanisms. It is found in abnormalities of the autonomic nervous system, the endocrine system, sinus nodal blood supply (such as in myocardial infarction), and in disease or damage to atrial muscle, as in amyloidosis, diffuse fibrosis, collagen disease, infection, and pericardial disease. It may also be caused by drugs (see below) and electrolyte disturbances. SA nodal dysfunction is often associated with AV nodal dysfunction.[4]

MANAGEMENT

1. Careful history-taking is needed to discover possible causes.
2. If a 12-lead ECG does not show the typical findings discussed above, a 24-hour Holter recording gives important information, since most patients with SSS have their symptoms intermittently.
3. Correct all possible causes such as by discontinuing possible offending drugs. If unsuccessful:
4. A pacemaker is indicated in symptomatic patients.

NOTE CAREFULLY

- Certain drugs will change latent SSS into manifest sinus dysfunction, among which are beta blockers, class IC drugs (flecainide, encainide, propafenone), amiodarone, class IA drugs (quinidine, procainamide, disopyramide), verapamil, diltiazem, lithium, and reserpine.
- Carotid sinus massage is often used on patients suspected of having carotid hypersensitivity as the cause of their symptoms. It is important to know, however, that carotid sinus massage may cause pauses of 6 sec or more in patients who are older than 65 years of age (but are otherwise asymptomatic).

SUMMARY

Slow atrial rhythms may be the result of sinus bradycardia, sinoatrial block, sinus arrest, or sick sinus syndrome. SA block is a disturbance in SA conduction, and sinus arrest is a disturbance in impulse formation in the sinus node. Both may result from infiltrative disease as well as excessive vagal stimulation, carotid hypersensitivity, myocardial infarction, acute myocarditis, drugs, and hyper- or hypokalemia.

In sick sinus syndrome, SA nodal dysfunction is frequently associated with AV nodal dysfunction, often the result of disease of atrial muscle and abnormalities of sinus node automaticity.

A systematic approach to the diagnosis of slow atrial rhythms requires a 12-lead ECG, which is evaluated for cause (for example, myocardial infarction) and mechanism of the bradycardia. In case of diminished cardiac output, atropine is given and temporary pacing may be necessary. Otherwise, no treatment is required.

References

1. Bethge, C., Gebhardt-Seehausen, U., and Mullges, W.: The human sinus nodal electrogram: Techniques and clinical results of intra-atrial recordings in patients with and without sick sinus syndrome. Am. Heart J. 112(5):1074–1082, 1986.
2. Pisapia, A., Leheuzey, J.Y., Faure, J., et al.: Sino-atrial dissociation: Evidence by intracardiac recordings in man and by microelectrode studies on isolated rabbit atrium. Pace 11(1):23–32, 1988.
3. Ferrer, M.T.: Sick sinus syndrome in atrial disease. J.A.M.A. 206:645, 1968.
4. Jordan, J.L., and Mandel, W.J.: Disorders of sinus function. In Mandel, W.J. (ed.): Cardiac Arrhythmias: Their Mechanisms, Diagnosis, and Management. Philadelphia, 1987, J.B. Lippincott, pp. 143–185.

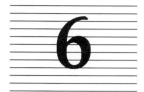

C H A P T E R

6

Atrioventricular Block

EMERGENCY APPROACH

Emergency situations requiring immediate intervention are frequently encountered in the setting of complete atrioventricular (AV) block (third degree) with a broad QRS complex, in which case the immediate insertion of a pacemaker is commonly indicated. Lesser degrees of AV block are also covered in this chapter.

CLASSIFICATION OF ATRIOVENTRICULAR BLOCK

AV block is traditionally divided into first-, second-, and third-degree types. First-degree AV block has a prolonged PR interval with all P waves conducted; second-degree block shows P waves not conducted to the ventricle and is divided into type I, type II, and second-degree block with 2:1 conduction. In third-degree AV block there is no conduction between atrium and ventricle. Important in management is the width of the QRS complex (narrow or broad).

NONINVASIVE METHODS FOR DETERMINING SITE OF ATRIOVENTRICULAR BLOCK

In AV block the conduction defect may be located in the AV node, bundle of His, bundle branches, or any combination of these (Fig. 6–1).[1] Since AV nodal block has a better prognosis and treatment differs from that for subnodal block, determination of the location and type of block is important. In this regard, much can be learned on the surface ECG from the PR interval, QRS duration, and the response of the block to noninvasive interventions such as atropine, exercise, catecholamines, or vagal maneuvers (Table 6–1).

Interventions that slow AV conduction, such as vagal maneuvers, worsen AV nodal block, but, because the number of impulses passing through the AV node declines, they improve subnodal block. On the other

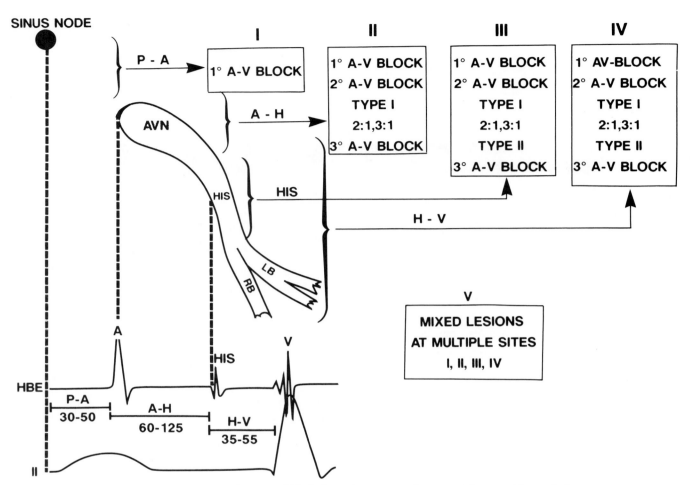

Figure 6–1. Location and types of block from the sinus node area to the ventricles and the corresponding measurements in the His bundle electrogram (HBE). In the left lower portion of the figure a His bundle electrogram and lead II tracing are schematically shown. The intervals noted are PA, AH, and HV; normal values are shown in milliseconds. *PA interval:* From the beginning of the P wave in the ECG to the atrial deflection (A) in the His bundle electrogram; *AH interval:* From the atrial deflection to the first deflection of the His bundle; corresponds to AV nodal transmission time; *HV interval:* From the onset of the His bundle deflection to the onset of the ventricular deflection in the His bundle electrogram, indicating the time required to travel from the bundle of His to the ventricles over the bundle branch system. (Modified from Narula, O.S., Scherlag, B.J., Samet, P., et al.: Atrioventricular block localization and classification by His bundle recordings. Am. J. Med. 50:146, 1971.)

Table 6–1. **Noninvasive Interventions to Determine Site of Atrioventricular Block; Effect on Atrioventricular Conduction**

Intervention	AV Nodal Conduction	Subnodal Conduction
Atropine	Improves	Worsens
Exercise or catecholamines	Improves	Worsens
Carotid sinus massage	Worsens	Improves

REST   **START EXERCISE**   **DURING EXERCISE**

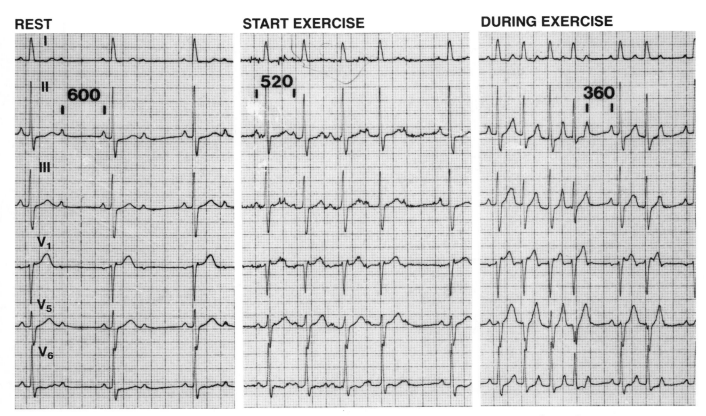

Figure 6–2. The left panel shows 2:1 AV block. AV nodal conduction improves with exercise. This indicates that the AV conduction disturbance is located in the AV node.

hand, interventions such as atropine and exercise improve AV nodal conduction (Fig. 6–2), but because of the increase in number of impulses conducted through the AV node, they worsen subnodal conduction problems. Thus, carotid sinus massage worsens AV nodal block and improves subnodal block; atropine, exercise, and catecholamines improve AV nodal block and worsen subnodal block.

HIS BUNDLE ELECTROGRAM

The His bundle electrogram is an intracardiac recording of the electrical activity in the atria, bundle of His, and ventricles.[2] The three complexes seen on a His bundle electrogram are depicted in Figure 6–1. The A wave represents low right atrial activation; the H deflection represents electrical activation of the His bundle; and the V deflection represents ventricular activation. The normal AH interval is 60 to 125 msec and the normal HV interval is 35 to 55 msec.

V₁

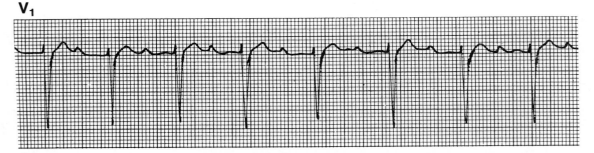

Figure 6–3. An example of a prolonged PR interval. A PR interval of 0.28 sec or more suggests AV nodal pathology.

PROLONGED PR INTERVAL

The PR interval reflects AV conduction time and is measured from the onset of the P wave to the beginning of the QRS complex. A prolonged PR interval (first-degree block) may be the result of conduction delay in the atrium, AV node, bundle of His, or bundle branches (Fig. 6–1). Although the actual site of delay cannot be determined by the surface ECG, a prolongation to 0.28 sec or more, such as in the PR seen in Figure 6–3, usually indicates AV nodal pathology.

An accurate measure of the site of delay in a prolonged PR interval can be obtained only by recording a His bundle electrogram. This will indicate whether the prolonged PR interval is based on an AV nodal conduction delay, a subnodal conduction problem (HV longer than 55 msec), or both.

SECOND-DEGREE ATRIOVENTRICULAR BLOCK

Second-degree AV block is divided into:[3]

> Type I (AV Wenckebach or Mobitz I)
> Type II (Mobitz II)
> 2:1 AV block

In second-degree AV block some of the sinus impulses are not conducted to the ventricles. The pathology may be either in the AV node or within or below the bundle of His, each with different clinical implications, treatment, and prognosis. A QRS duration of less than 0.12 sec indicates that the block is in the AV node or in the bundle of His. When a QRS of 0.12 sec or longer is present, apart from block in the bundle branch system, additional block can be located in the AV node or bundle of His. In type I AV block the QRS can be narrow or wide. The PR before the nonconducted beat is longer than the PR of the sinus impulse that follows the pause. In type II AV block the PR intervals are identical and the QRS is wide, unless the conduction disturbance is located in the bundle of His.

TYPE I ATRIOVENTRICULAR BLOCK
(AV WENCKEBACH)

ECG RECOGNITION

P Waves. Sinus.

PR Intervals. Lengthen progressively before the dropped beat.

QRS. Narrow or wide.

Rhythm. Group beating.

R-R Intervals. Shorten because the largest increment in the PR interval is usually between the first and second PR interval; however, the pattern may be atypical. Pauses are less than twice the shortest cycle.

Conduction. Improves with atropine, exercise, or catecholamines, and worsens with carotid sinus massage when the impairment in conduction is in the AV node (Table 6–1).

An example of 3:2 AV Wenckebach is given in Figure 6–4; of every three P waves only two are conducted. Note the group beating and lengthening of the second PR interval of each group; the third P wave is not conducted.

CLINICAL IMPLICATIONS

In type I AV block the conduction problem is usually at the level of the AV node, and it can be caused by acute inferior wall myocardial infarction (MI), digitalis toxicity, acute myocarditis, drugs, old age, or following open heart surgery.

In acute inferior wall MI the development of AV conduction problems can frequently be anticipated when there is ST elevation in lead V_4R indicating an occlusion proximally in the right coronary artery. Approximately 45 percent of such patients develop second-degree or complete AV block, placing them at 2½ times the risk of those who do not develop block.

Chronic second-degree AV nodal block is usually benign in patients without organic heart disease. However, when there is organic heart disease the prognosis is related to the underlying disease.

MANAGEMENT

In acute inferior wall MI, AV conduction problems are transient and usually require only observation. Approximately one-half of the type I AV blocks associated with acute inferior wall MI progress to complete AV block. If complete AV block develops secondary to inferior wall MI, the escape pacemaker is usually a dependable AV junctional rhythm and the patient may require observation only.

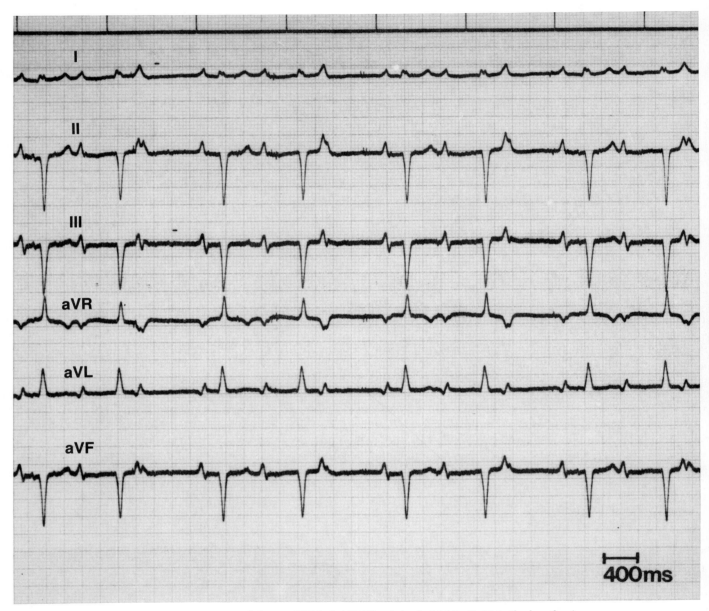

Figure 6–4. Type I second-degree AV block (AV Wenckebach, Mobitz I). Note the lengthening PR intervals, blocked P waves, and group beating.

TYPE II ATRIOVENTRICULAR BLOCK

ECG RECOGNITION

P Waves. Sinus.

PR Intervals. Normal or slightly prolonged and the same before and after the nonconducted P wave.

QRS. Broad (0.12 sec or more) unless intra-His block is present.

Rhythm. Ventricular rhythm irregular because of nonconducted beats.

Conduction. Worsens with atropine, exercise, or catecholamines, but may improve when carotid sinus massage slows sinus rhythm. The typical ECG of type II AV block is illustrated in Figure 6–5. Note the nonconducted sinus P waves, the fixed PR throughout the tracing, and the broad QRS—all hallmarks of type II AV block. The PR interval is slightly prolonged.

MECHANISM

The lesion in type II AV block is either located in the bundle of His or involves both bundle branches, one completely and the other intermittently.

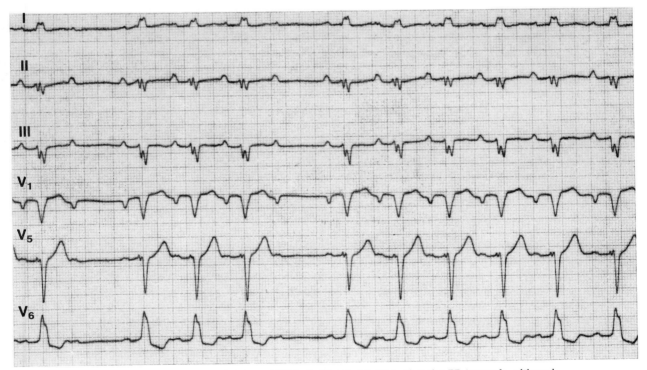

Figure 6–5. Type II second-degree AV block (Mobitz II). Note that the PR intervals, although prolonged, are identical before and after the dropped beat. The QRS is broad with a typical left bundle branch block configuration, indicating that the Mobitz II block is located in the right bundle branch.

The persistent block of one bundle causes the ventricular complexes to be broad; intermittent block of the other bundle causes nonconducted beats. The most common cause of type II AV block is chronic fibrotic disease of the conduction system in the elderly; it may also occur in anteroseptal myocardial infarction.

CLINICAL IMPLICATIONS

Type II AV block is not as common as type I. It is associated with chronic fibrotic disease of the conduction system or anteroseptal MI, is often accompanied by syncope, and may progress to complete heart block with a slow ventricular escape rhythm.

MANAGEMENT

Type II AV block associated with syncope requires the insertion of a temporary pacemaker followed by a permanent one in patients with chronic fibrotic disease of the conduction system. In patients with anteroseptal MI and syncope, complete block is usually temporary, and (if the patient survives the acute stage of MI) implantation of a permanent pacemaker is rarely needed.

2:1 ATRIOVENTRICULAR BLOCK

ECG RECOGNITION

P Waves. Sinus.

PR Intervals. Normal or prolonged.

QRS. Narrow if the conduction problem is in the AV node or His bundle; broad in case of bundle branch pathology.

Rhythm. Regular.

R-R Intervals. Regular.

Conduction. In cases of AV nodal pathology, the block improves with atropine, exercise, or catecholamines and worsens with carotid sinus massage. In cases of subnodal pathology, the block worsens with atropine, exercise, or catecholamines and may improve when sinus rate slows with carotid sinus massage.

In Figure 6–6 there is 1:1 AV conduction with a normal PR interval at rest at a sinus rate of 65 beats per minute. During exercise, when the sinus rate accelerates to 145 beats per minute, the conduction ratio deteriorates to 3:1. The worsening of AV block during exercise indicates a subnodal lesion (Table 6–1).

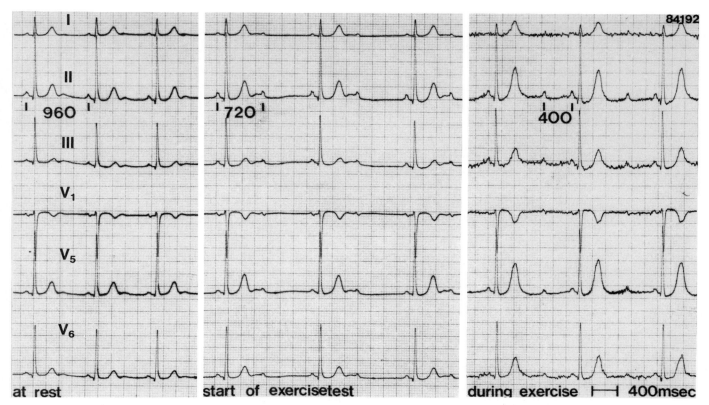

Figure 6–6. When the patient is at rest there is sinus rhythm with a normal PR interval. However, during exercise a high-degree AV block develops in this patient with a narrow QRS complex. This sequence of events indicates that the block must be in the bundle of His (see text).

CLINICAL IMPLICATIONS

The clinical implications of 2:1 AV block depend upon the site of pathology (AV nodal or subnodal). The level of block can be determined by noninvasive methods (Table 6–1) or by a His bundle electrogram (Fig. 6–1). In acute inferior wall MI, although the block may become complete, a pacemaker is usually not necessary. In acute anterior wall MI a temporary pacemaker may be indicated if the QRS is broad and the condition is accompanied by syncope or hemodynamic deterioration.

COMPLETE ATRIOVENTRICULAR BLOCK (THIRD-DEGREE AV BLOCK)

ECG RECOGNITION

P Waves. Sinus.

P/QRS Relationship. None (AV dissociation).

QRS. Narrow if the site of block is in the AV node and the escape rhythm originates in the AV junction; broad if the escape rhythm occurs in the ventricle or in the AV junction in the presence of bundle branch block.

Rate. Less than 50 beats per minute with the exception of congenital AV block, where the rate may be higher.

Rhythm. AV dissociation (regular sinus rhythm; regular ventricular rhythm).

Figure 6–7 shows 2:1 AV block and the sudden onset of complete AV block in a patient with anteroseptal MI, right bundle branch block, and left posterior hemiblock. The QRS configuration of the conducted beats at the beginning of the tracings shows right bundle branch block; the right axis deviation is the result of left posterior hemiblock. When third-degree AV block suddenly occurs (after the fourth QRS complex) the morphology of the escape ventricular rhythm is that of a focus in the left posterior fascicle. Note that the QRS complexes in lead V_1 still show right bundle branch block

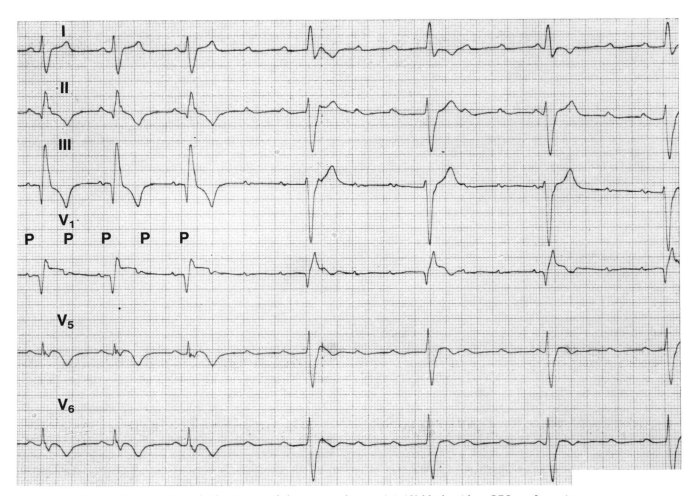

Figure 6–7. At the beginning of the tracing there is 2:1 AV block with a QRS configuration indicating block in the posterior fascicle and in the right bundle branch. This suddenly changes into complete AV block with an escape rhythm arising in the left posterior fascicle (see text).

configuration, reflecting a focus in the left bundle branch; the left axis deviation indicates impulse formation in the posterior fascicle.

Sudden onset of complete AV block may also occur after a PVC or a paced beat in a patient with bundle branch block and hemiblock. The most likely mechanism is induction of phase 4 block in the only remaining fascicle that was still able to conduct before the pause.[4] The first three complexes in Figure 6–8 show right bundle branch block and left anterior hemiblock. A spontaneously occurring ventricular premature beat (fourth QRS complex) causes a pause during which the fibers in the left posterior fascicle are depolarizing (phase 4 depolarization); that is, they are becoming less and less negative and are therefore losing their capability to conduct. By the time the first sinus beat arrives following the ventricular premature beat, conduction is no longer possible in the posterior fascicle of the left bundle branch and was already blocked in the anterior fascicle. Complete AV block persists for almost 5 seconds and is terminated by an escape beat from the left bundle branch.

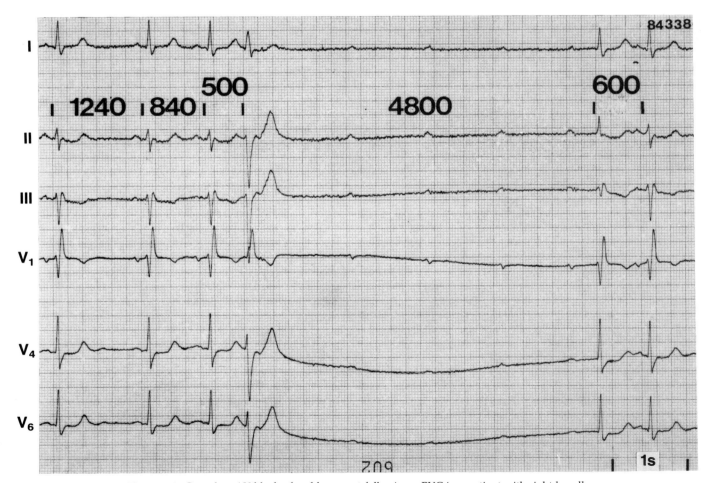

Figure 6–8. Complete AV block of sudden onset following a PVC in a patient with right bundle branch block and left anterior hemiblock. The most likely mechanism is induction of phase 4 block in the only remaining fascicle that was still able to conduct before the pause (the posterior fascicle).

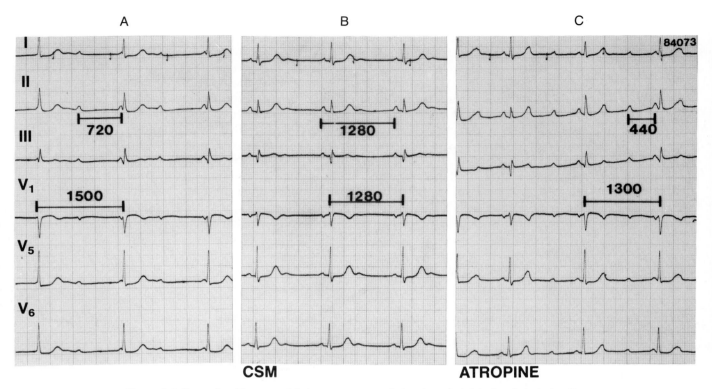

Figure 6–9. Example of how carotid sinus massage and atropine administration help in locating the site of block in a patient with complete AV block with a narrow QRS. As shown, slowing of the sinus node by carotid massage improves AV nodal conduction, whereas atropine worsens conduction. This indicates that the conduction abnormality is located in the bundle of His.

Figure 6–9A is an example of third-degree AV block with a narrow QRS complex. The level of block could therefore be either AV nodal or within the bundle of His. In Figure 6–9B, carotid sinus massage (CSM) depresses AV nodal conduction and 1:1 conduction ensues because of sinus slowing, proving that the AV node is not involved. In Figure 6–9C, when atropine is given to increase the rate of the sinus node and to shorten AV nodal conduction time, high-degree AV block is seen. These observations indicate that the lesion is in the bundle of His and not in the AV node.

CLINICAL IMPLICATIONS

In complete AV block the rate and dependability of the ventricular rhythm are related to the level of the lesion and the rate of the escape rhythm. In general, the dependability of the escape rhythm is better the higher its location in the conduction system.

MANAGEMENT

Complete AV block with a broad QRS usually requires the insertion of a pacemaker. If the QRS is narrow, no immediate treatment is necessary. In such case, one should determine the cause of the block and then make a judgment regarding the necessity of pacemaker insertion.

ALTERNATING BUNDLE BRANCH BLOCK

Among patients with bundle branch block (see Chapter 1), those at highest risk to develop complete AV block are patients having alternating bundle branch block. In such cases, during sinus rhythm one bundle branch block pattern (e.g., left bundle branch block) suddenly changes into another pattern of bundle branch block (e.g., right bundle branch block). As shown in Figures 6–10 and 6–11, that finding implies severe conduction abnormalities

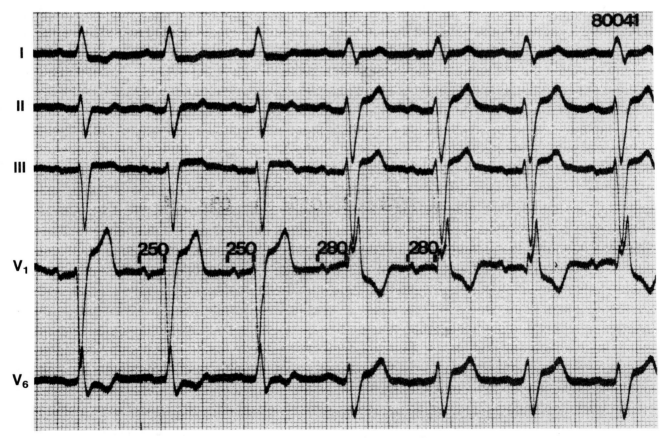

Figure 6–10. Example of alternating bundle branch block. The left part of the figure shows sinus rhythm with left bundle branch block and a PR interval of 250 msec. This suddenly changes into right bundle branch block with a PR interval of 280 msec.

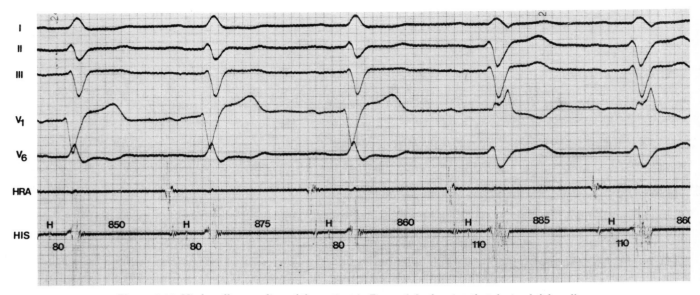

Figure 6–11. His bundle recording of the patient in Figure 6–9, showing that during left bundle branch block an HV interval of 80 msec suddenly prolongs to 110 msec with the appearance of right bundle branch block.

in both bundle branches and indicates the necessity for implantation of a permanent pacemaker.

SUMMARY

First-degree AV block has a prolonged PR interval with all beats conducted; second-degree block has dropped beats and is divided into type I, type II, and second-degree block with 2:1 conduction. Third-degree AV block is classified according to the QRS width, narrow or broad, a feature that helps to determine management. Knowledge of the level of the pathology in the AV conduction system is of importance to determine prognosis and management. This can be assessed noninvasively by observing AV conduction on the ECG in response to atropine, carotid sinus massage, and exercise. Immediate pacemaker insertion is usually indicated only in complete (third-degree) AV block with a broad QRS complex.

References

1. Narula, O.S.: Atrioventricular block. In Narula, O.S.: Cardiac Arrhythmias: Electrophysiology, Diagnosis and Management. Baltimore, 1979, Williams & Wilkins, pp. 85–113.
2. Scherlag, B.J., Lau, S.H., Helfant, R.H., et al.: Catheter technique for recording His bundle activity in man. Circulation 39:13, 1969.
3. Puech, P., Grolleau, R., and Guimond, C.: Incidence of different types of A-V block and their location by His bundle recordings. In Wellens, H.J.J., Lie, K.I., and Janse, M.J. (eds.): The Conduction System of the Heart. Leiden, 1976, H.E. Stenfert Kroese BV.
4. Rosenbaum, M.B., Elizari, M.V., Levi, R.J., et al.: Paroxysmal atrioventricular block related to hypopolarization and spontaneous diastolic depolarization. Chest 63:678, 1973.

C H A P T E R

7

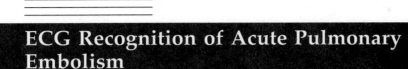

ECG Recognition of Acute Pulmonary Embolism

EMERGENCY APPROACH

EXAMINE THE ECG FOR
- Rhythm disturbances
- A shift in the axis to the right in comparison with the ECG prior to the acute event (need not be outside the normal range of +90 to −30 degrees)
- Appearance of a right bundle branch block (RBBB) pattern
- Pseudoinfarction patterns

Sudden changes in the ECG suggesting pulmonary embolism call for an emergency echocardiogram.

THERAPY
- Oxygen
- Analgesics
- Full-dose heparin
- Thrombolytic therapy

PREVENTION

Avoid Venous Stasis

Early mobilization and ambulation when possible
External compression of the legs for patients on complete bedrest.

Anticoagulants

If heart failure is present or the patient is on long-term bedrest

PATHOPHYSIOLOGY OF ACUTE PULMONARY EMBOLISM

Acute pulmonary embolism is the sudden obstruction of a central and/or peripheral pulmonary artery. If such an obstruction is significant, it results

129

in acute pulmonary hypertension, right-sided dilatation and clockwise cardiac rotation, right ventricular failure, marked ventilation-perfusion disturbance, and acute lowering of the cardiac output. This leads to sudden severe dyspnea, chest pain, and sometimes syncope.

VALUE OF THE ECG

Pulmonary embolism is commonly overlooked and often fatal. If the acute phase is recognized and treated appropriately, death can be prevented in 75 percent of patients who otherwise would have died.

The ECG signs of acute pulmonary embolism are not 100 percent diagnostic, and prior cardiac disease may make these ECG signs even less specific and less obvious.[1] However, certain ECG findings can cause the informed examiner to have a high degree of suspicion, in which case the diagnosis can be confirmed by an emergency echocardiogram. The echocardiogram sensitively reflects the right ventricular pressure and volume overload of acute pulmonary embolism and is quite useful for this often difficult diagnosis.[2, 3]

When acute pulmonary embolism is suspected, serial tracings are necessary because although sudden dilatation of the right ventricle and elevated right-sided pressures are usually accompanied by dynamic ECG changes, a single ECG may show no obvious signs of pulmonary embolism, whereas the changes may be apparent on subsequent tracings.

COMMON ECG FINDINGS IN THE ACUTE PHASE

The common ECG findings in the acute phase of pulmonary embolism (Table 7–1) consist of arrhythmias and abnormalities of the P wave, QRS complex, ST segment, and T wave.

Table 7–1. **ECG Findings in Acute Pulmonary Embolism**

Rhythm
  Sinus tachycardia
  Atrial fibrillation
  Atrial flutter
  Premature beats (right atrial, right ventricular)
  Ventricular fibrillation
P waves
  Right axis deviation
QRS complex
  Axis shift (usually to the right)
  RBBB pattern
  Q waves in leads V_1, III, and aVF
  S waves in leads I and aVL
  Clockwise rotation of the heart
ST-T
  ST segment elevation in leads V_1, aVR, and III
  Symmetrical T wave inversion in precordial
    leads V_1–V_5 (subacute phase)
  T wave negativity in leads III and aVF
    (subacute phase)

ARRHYTHMIAS

Arrhythmias associated with acute pulmonary embolism are the result of right ventricular failure and acute dilatation of the right atrium and right ventricle. They are:

Sinus tachycardia
Atrial fibrillation
Atrial flutter
Right atrial premature beats
Right ventricular premature beats

P WAVE ABNORMALITIES

P wave changes, when present in acute pulmonary embolism, are those of right axis deviation and right atrial enlargement (P-pulmonale), for example, tall P waves (>2.5 mm) in leads II, III, and aVF.

QRS COMPLEX ABNORMALITIES

Axis. In the frontal plane, the QRS axis usually shifts to the right of the axis in the pre-embolic state. Such an axis shift does not have to be in the abnormal range, although on occasion there may be frank right axis deviation of more than +90 degrees.

Right Ventricular Conduction Delay. In acute pulmonary embolism there is often an abrupt appearance of RBBB pattern because of acute stretching of that bundle branch when the right heart abruptly dilates. This is reflected by an ECG pattern of incomplete or complete RBBB.

Normally the right ventricle contributes little to the QRS complex so that the sudden appearance and growth of a late R wave in lead V_1 is an important sign of acute pulmonary embolism, especially when combined with ST elevation and a positive T wave in that lead. In patients with no pre-existing heart disease, the completeness of the RBBB pattern correlates with the percentage of pulmonary blood flow blocked by the embolus. When the pattern is that of complete RBBB (QRS >0.11 sec), there is 50 percent or more occlusion of the pulmonary circulation.

Secondary to the delayed activation of the right ventricle is the appearance of S waves in leads I and aVL. Because of clockwise rotation of the heart, Q waves appear in leads III and aVF—a finding that is often misdiagnosed as acute inferior wall myocardial infarction.

ST SEGMENT ELEVATION

ST segment elevation may be seen in leads V_1 and aVR; both leads reflect right-sided dilatation. The ST segment elevation in lead V_1 is an early sign, and when associated with RBBB pattern and a positive T wave in that lead it should immediately raise the suspicion of pulmonary embolism. Such a pattern differs from that of uncomplicated RBBB in which the ST segment is not elevated and the T wave is opposite in polarity to the QRS.

T WAVE ABNORMALITIES

Symmetrical T wave negativity in the precordial leads usually develops within 24 to 48 hours following the acute event and may persist for several weeks.

CLOCKWISE ROTATION

The clockwise rotation of the heart that is seen in acute pulmonary embolism is the result of the sudden right-sided dilatation and pressure elevation. This is reflected in the ECG by a shift in the transitional zone (equiphasic complex) to the left.

Normally in the precordial leads the transition from mostly negative to mostly positive occurs at lead V_3 or V_4. In acute pulmonary embolism, this transition takes place more to the left at lead V_5 and sometimes even at lead V_6. When this occurs, clockwise rotation of the heart is said to be present. Normal and abnormal transitional zones are illustrated in Figure 7–1.

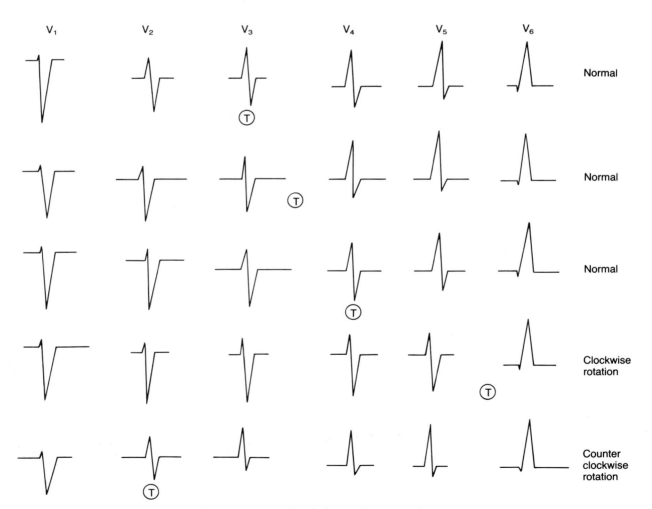

Figure 7–1. Normal and abnormal transitional zones.

ABNORMAL Q AND/OR S WAVES

Since in acute pulmonary embolism the right precordial leads record an intracavitary complex over a dilated right atrium, QS complexes may appear in lead V_1. When this pattern is associated with Q waves in leads III and aVF, one should very carefully rule out pulmonary embolism.

In Figure 7–2, the pre-embolic ECG should be compared with that in the acute phase of pulmonary embolism. Note the development of sinus tachycardia and all of the signs of acute dilatation of the right heart (i.e., RBBB pattern, slight ST elevation in leads V_1 and aVR, a shift of the QRS axis from 0 degrees to +30 degrees, the development of Q waves in leads

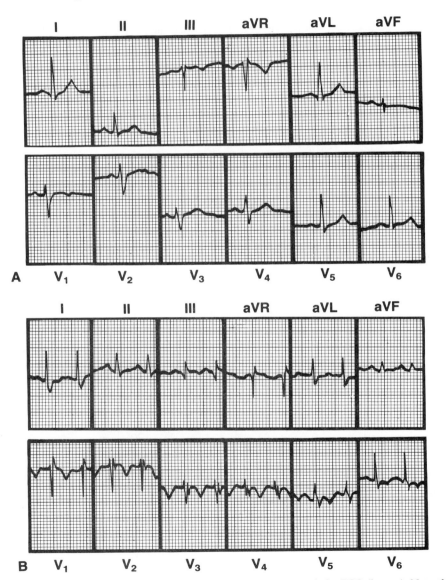

Figure 7–2. The pre-embolic ECG *(top)* compared with the postembolic ECG *(bottom)*. Note the development of sinus tachycardia, right bundle branch block, a shift in the QRS axis from 0 degrees to +30 degrees, and S waves in leads I and aVL and Q waves in leads III and aVF. The T wave is inverted and symmetrical in the precordial leads.

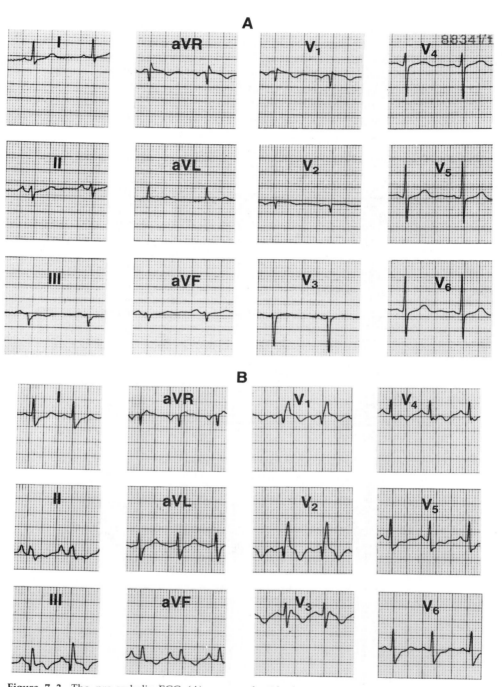

Figure 7–3. The pre-embolic ECG (A) compared with the postembolic ECG (B). Note the development of sinus tachycardia, right bundle branch block pattern, a shift in the QRS axis from −45 degrees to +90 degrees, and S waves in leads I and aVL and Q waves in lead III. There are ST segment elevation in leads V_1 and aVR and T wave inversion in leads V_1 to V_4.

III and aVF, the development of S waves in leads I and aVL, and clockwise rotation of the heart). Note that the transitional zone (equiphasic deflection) shifts from lead V_4 in the pre-embolic ECG to lead V_5 in the postembolic tracing.

Figure 7–3 is another example of the pre-embolic compared with the postembolic state. In the pre-embolic state, this patient had a left axis deviation, which shifted to the right (+85 degrees). Note the development of sinus tachycardia, a deep S wave in leads I and aVL, a Q wave in lead III, an RBBB pattern, and elevated ST segments in leads aVR and V_1.

The two tracings in Figure 7–4 are from patients in the acute phase of pulmonary embolism. All show the typical pattern of acute pulmonary embolism.

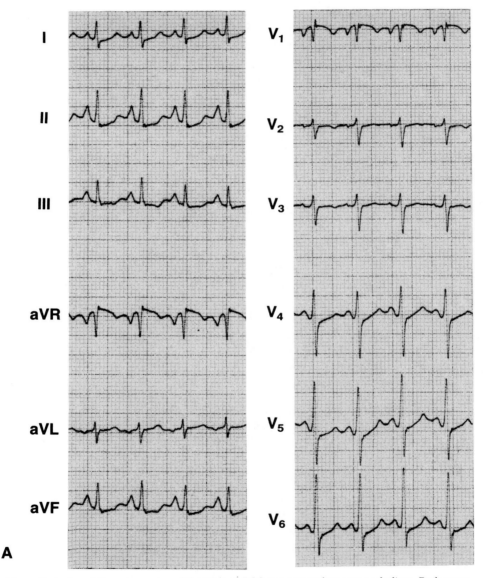

Figure 7–4. *A* and *B* are examples of the 12-lead ECG in acute pulmonary embolism. Both cases show sinus tachycardia, right bundle branch block pattern, S wave in leads I and aVL, elevated ST segments in leads V_1 and aVR, and clockwise rotation of the heart.

Illustration continued on following page

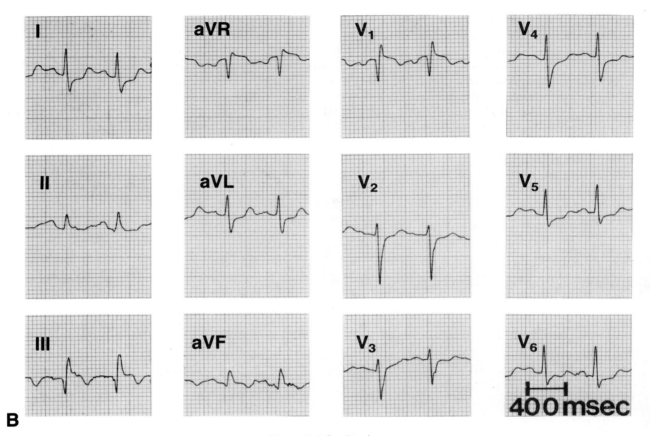

B

Figure 7–4 *Continued*

SUBACUTE PHASE FOLLOWING SPONTANEOUS RESOLUTION OF THE CLOT OR THROMBOLYTIC THERAPY

The ECG pattern in the subacute phase of pulmonary embolism (Table 7–1) depends upon the moment when the tracing is recorded in the evolving course of the pathology. Serial ECG recordings may show resolution of the right ventricular conduction delay and the axis shift and development of deep T wave inversion in the precordial leads up to leads V_5 and V_6 and in leads III and aVF; these T wave changes may persist for weeks.

CHRONIC PHASE

The ECG during the chronic phase of pulmonary embolism depends on the dissolution of the clot. There may be residual evidence of right atrial and right ventricular hypertrophy.

DIFFERENTIAL DIAGNOSIS

DISTINGUISHING MYOCARDIAL INFARCTION FROM ACUTE PULMONARY EMBOLISM

Acute massive pulmonary embolism involving the main pulmonary arteries may simulate myocardial infarction, especially since both conditions are associated with a fall in cardiac output, abnormal Q waves, ST segment elevation, and T wave changes. For example, right axis deviation, with Q waves and T wave changes in the inferior leads, may mimic inferior wall myocardial infarction. Although the RBBB pattern and ST segment elevation in lead V_1 should make one suspicious of pulmonary embolism, this pattern is also seen when acute anteroseptal infarction is complicated by RBBB. Several differences help in the diagnosis, although none are truly specific.

In acute pulmonary embolism:

1. The acute shortness of breath is more pronounced than would be expected in myocardial infarction.
2. The ECG, although abnormal, is not typical for myocardial infarction. For example, the presence of both inferior wall and anterior wall myocardial infarction may be suggested in one 12-lead ECG (i.e., Q waves may be seen in leads III and aVF, but not in lead II, and these may be associated with a QR pattern in lead V_1).
3. The chest roentgenogram does not show pulmonary congestion, although there is severe dyspnea.
4. The diagnostic usefulness of the ECG is enhanced when combined with echocardiography.

SIGNS AND SYMPTOMS

The physical signs and symptoms of acute pulmonary embolism relate to a decrease in pulmonary blood flow with its attendant decrease in oxygen exchange in the affected zone and eventual decrease in cardiac output. They are:

1. Hypoxemia, hyperventilation, dyspnea, and apprehension.
2. Confusion, syncope, or shock may result if the decrease in cardiac output is severe.
3. If there is pulmonary infarction, there may be hemoptysis, and the patient may experience pleuritic chest pain.

Note. In a patient on bedrest, one should be alerted to the possibility of pulmonary embolism when there are unexplained fever, dyspnea, tachypnea, and tachycardia.

PHYSICAL FINDINGS

Physical findings are related to right ventricular hypertension, right ventricular failure, and the increase in pulmonary artery pressure. Right ventricular hypertension can result in a palpable right ventricular impulse, an increase in "a" waves in the jugular venous pulse, and an audible right ventricular S4. Right ventricular failure can cause tachycardia, an increase in jugular venous distention, tricuspid regurgitation, an S3 heart sound, and hepatomegaly. The increased pulmonary artery pressure can produce a palpable pulmonary artery pulsation, splitting of S2 with an exaggerated P2, and a pulmonary ejection murmur.

TREATMENT

1. Oxygen
2. Analgesics
3. Full-dose heparin[4]
4. Thrombolytic therapy[5-7]

PREVENTION

Every effort should be made to prevent acute pulmonary embolism by encouraging early ambulation or mobilization when possible and by employing external compression of the legs for patients on complete bedrest. Anticoagulants may be indicated for patients with heart failure or those on long-term bedrest.

SUMMARY

The ECG changes associated with acute pulmonary embolism are due to acute right ventricular dilatation. These changes, which begin abruptly, require serial ECG tracings. Rhythm disturbances, axis shifts, the sudden appearance of a right ventricular conduction delay, a Q wave in lead III, an S wave in lead I, and pseudoinfarction patterns may develop.

References

1. Brugada, P., Gorgels, A.P., and Wellens, H.J.J.: The electrocardiogram in pulmonary embolism. In Wellens, H.J.J., and Kulbertus, H.E.: What's New in Electrocardiography. The Hague, 1981, Martinus Nijhoff, p. 366.
2. Come, P.C.: Echocardiographic recognition of pulmonary arterial disease and determination of its cause. Am. J. Med. 84(3,1):384–394, 1988.
3. Jardin, F., Dubourg, O., Gueret, P., et al.: Quantitative two-dimensional echocardiography in massive pulmonary embolism: Emphasis on ventricular interdependence and leftward septal displacement. J. Am. Coll. Cardiol. 10(6):1201–1206, 1987.
4. Raskob, G.E., Carter, C.J., and Hull, R.D.: Heparin therapy for venous thrombosis and pulmonary embolism. Blood Rev. 2(4):251–258, 1988.
5. Tissue plasminogen activator for the treatment of acute pulmonary embolism. A collaborative study by the PIOPED Investigators. Chest 97(3):528–533, 1990.
6. Verstraete, M., Miller, G.A., Bounameaux, H., et al.: Intravenous and intrapulmonary recombinant tissue-type plasminogen activator in the treatment of acute massive pulmonary embolism. Circulation 77(2):353–360, 1988.
7. Goldhaber, S.Z., Meyerovitz, M.F., Markis, J.E., et al.: Thrombolytic therapy of acute pulmonary embolism: Current status and future potential. J. Am. Coll. Cardiol. 10(5, Suppl. B):96B–104B, 1987.

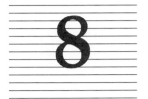

CHAPTER

8

Digitalis-Induced Emergencies

SYSTEMATIC DIAGNOSTIC APPROACH

1. Obtain periodic 12-lead ECGs on all patients in your care taking digitalis.
2. Question the patient regarding noncardiac signs of digitalis toxicity and concomitant medication that may interact with digitalis.
3. Know the ECG signs of digitalis dysrhythmias.
4. Look specifically for bradycardia, tachycardia, inappropriate regularity (such as in atrial fibrillation or flutter), or group beating.

EMERGENCY MANAGEMENT

1. Discontinue digitalis.
2. Bedrest (no sympathetic stimulation!)
3. Continuous ECG monitoring
4. If hemodynamically unstable, phenytoin is indicated unless digitalis antibodies are available.
5. Ventricular pacing is indicated:
   - In symptomatic bradycardia
   - During treatment with phenytoin because suppression of the tachycardia may be followed by asystole
6. Correct potassium and magnesium deficits.

AVOID

1. Sympathetic stimulation (stress, anxiety, exercise, sympathomimetic drugs)
2. Carotid sinus massage
3. Fast or sudden cessation of pacing

INTRODUCTION

The emergencies created by digitalis are frequently not apparent to the casual observer or to the uninformed medical professional. Nonetheless, diagnosis and correct management are critical because of the high mortality associated with unrecognized and/or poorly managed cases of digitalis toxicity.[1] In fact, even the mortality itself, although unacceptably high, is often unacknowledged; the patient is said to have simply passed away because of a "bad heart." Because of this and because of the significant number of regular users of digitalis seen in hospitals and physicians' offices, all physicians who look after patients on digitalis and all emergency department and critical care professionals should be familiar with the mechanism, diagnosis, and treatment of digitalis dysrhythmias.

MECHANISM

The arrhythmias of digitalis toxicity are the result of (1) a block in conduction, which may be located in the sinoatrial [SA] and/or atrioventricular [AV] nodal regions, and/or (2) rapid impulse formation in the atrium, AV junction, and ventricular Purkinje system. Digitalis inhibits the enzyme sodium-potassium adenosinetriphosphatase (ATPase)[2] and thus interferes with the sodium pump, causing sodium to accumulate within the cell, which in turn alters the sodium-calcium exchange. This results in a buildup of calcium within the cell, a fact that explains the positive inotropic effect of the drug.[2] In an effort to rid the cell of excess calcium, after full repolarization (end of phase 3 of the action potential) there is a transient inward sodium current that briefly reduces the membrane potential (makes it less negative). It is this sodium current that causes the delayed afterdepolarization, which upon reaching threshold potential results in a propagated action potential called "triggered activity."[3] The mechanism of abnormal impulse formation in digitalis intoxication is the perpetuation of triggered activity in the atrium, AV junction, or the Purkinje system of the ventricles.[3]

Figure 8–1 illustrates the delayed afterdepolarization. The action potential in Figure 8–1A is followed by hyperpolarization of the membrane (marked negativity; *dark arrow* in Fig. 8–1A) and then a delayed afterdepolarization (*open arrow* in Fig. 8–1A), which in this case does not reach threshold potential. In Figure 8–1B the delayed afterdepolarization reaches threshold potential and results in triggered activity. Two factors that are known to cause delayed afterdepolarizations to reach threshold are catecholamines (sympathetic stimulation) and a shortening of the basic cycle length of the cardiac rhythm. As the cycle length of the basic rhythm increases, so does that of the triggered rhythm.[3, 4]

Conditions that may promote arrhythmic expressions of digitalis intoxication are increased sympathetic stimulation, which induces intracellular calcium overload; hypokalemia; hypercalcemia; hypomagnesemia; diuretics; ischemia and reperfusion; increased wall tension; and heart failure, all of which are of themselves capable of producing triggered activity.[5]

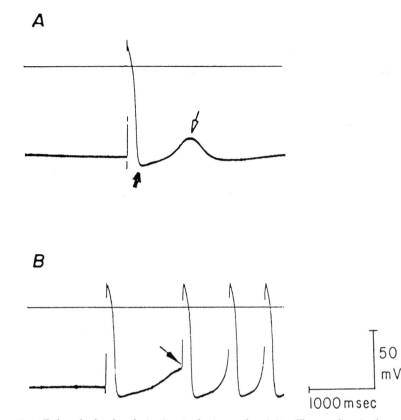

Figure 8–1. Delayed afterdepolarization and triggered activity. The top line is the reference 0 potential. (*A*) A driven action potential is followed by hyperpolarization (*solid arrow*) and then delayed afterdepolarization (*open arrow*). (*B*) A driven action potential is followed by a delayed afterdepolarization that reaches threshold potential. Nondriven action potentials (*arrow*) arise from the peak of each subsequent delayed afterdepolarization. (Modified from Wit, A.L., Boyden, P.A., Gadsby, D.C., and Cranefield, P.F.: Triggered activity as a cause of atrial arrhythmias. In Narula, O.S. (ed.): Cardiac Arrhythmias: Electrophysiology, Diagnosis, and Management. © 1979, the Williams & Wilkins Co., Baltimore.)

Suppressants of triggered activity are beta blockers, calcium antagonists, phenytoin, and caffeine.

MORTALITY IN UNDIAGNOSED DIGITALIS TOXICITY

The mortality following unrecognized digitalis dysrhythmias has been shown to be very high.[1] In the patients studied, when atrial tachycardia with block went unrecognized and digitalis was continued, 100 percent (7 of 7 patients) died; when the drug was stopped there was a 6 percent mortality (1 of 16 patients). When junctional tachycardia was not recognized as a digitalis dysrhythmia, 81 percent died (25 of 31 patients); when the diagnosis was made and the drug stopped, the mortality was 16 percent (7 of 43 patients).

FACTORS AFFECTING DOSAGE REQUIREMENTS IN PATIENTS TAKING DIGITALIS

DRUG INTERACTION

Digitalis dysrhythmias may result from interaction with other drugs that the patient is taking and other factors. These factors are summarized in Table 8–1. We have selected from this table some frequently prescribed cardioactive drugs that need a somewhat larger discussion.

Quinidine

When quinidine is added to digoxin therapy, the dose of digoxin should be decreased by approximately 50 percent. When quinidine is given to patients receiving digoxin, the serum digoxin concentration increases because of a reduction in digoxin volume of distribution and a decrease in renal and nonrenal clearance of digoxin.[7]

Amiodarone

Depending upon the dose, amiodarone increases plasma digoxin concentration due in part to a decrease in renal and nonrenal clearance of digoxin and in part to an increase in half-life.[7]

Table 8–1. **Factors Influencing Dosage Requirements in Patients Receiving Digitalis**

Factor	Higher Dosage Needed	Lower Dosage Needed
Intestinal resorption	Malabsorption Antacids Oral antibiotics Cholestyramine Cholestipol	Anticholinergic drugs
Body clearance (renal and nonrenal)	Hyperthyroidism	Renal disease Old age Hypothyroidism Quinidine Amiodarone Spirolactone Verapamil Diltiazem
Volume of distribution	Hyperthyroidism	Small people Old age Renal disease Hypothyroidism Chronic pulmonary disease Quinidine Spironolactone
Binding to cardiac muscle	Hyperkalemia Reserpine	Hypokalemia Hypomagnesemia
Unexplained sensitivity and/or tolerance	Young age Hypocalcemia	Congestive heart failure Myocardial ischemia Chronic pulmonary disease Hypercalcemia

Verapamil

Both renal and nonrenal clearance of digoxin decrease when digoxin and verapamil are combined. This effect develops gradually during the first few days and reaches a steady state within 7 days.[8]

Diltiazem

A 22 percent increase in steady-state plasma digoxin concentration occurs when diltiazem 180 mg/day is added to digoxin.

Note: Drugs that do not appear to affect digoxin concentration are procainamide, disopyramide, mexiletine, flecainide, ethmozine, and nifedipine.

TYPICAL DIGITALIS DYSRHYTHMIAS

Enhanced impulse formation, based on triggered activity and typical of digitalis toxicity, is located in the atria (frequently close to the sinus node), the AV junction, and in the His-Purkinje system. Common digitalis dysrhythmias are atrial tachycardia,[6] junctional tachycardia (including accelerated junctional rhythm),[6, 9] fascicular ventricular tachycardia (VT; including bidirectional VT),[6] and ventricular bigeminy. Digitalis also causes SA and AV block and suppresses phase 4 depolarization in normal pacemaker cells. It is important to know that in the healthy heart digitalis excess (e.g., as in a suicide attempt) results in conduction abnormalities only, whereas in the sick heart both conduction abnormalities and enhanced impulse formation occur.[10]

ECG RECOGNITION OF DIGITALIS DYSRHYTHMIAS

When caring for patients who are taking digitalis, be alert for four features:[10]

1. Bradycardia when the heart rate was previously normal or fast (caused by SA and/or AV block)
2. Tachycardia when the rate was previously normal (causes: atrial tachycardia, AV junctional tachycardia, fascicular ventricular tachycardia)
3. Unexpected rhythm regularity in a patient known to have an irregular rhythm (caused by complete AV block with a regular AV junctional rhythm in the patient with atrial fibrillation or atrial flutter)
4. Regular rhythm irregularity, such as the group beating of ventricular bigeminy, SA or AV Wenckebach, or combinations of these.

ATRIAL TACHYCARDIA WITH BLOCK

The ECG features of atrial tachycardia due to digitalis toxicity are:

1. Atrial rate is 130 to 250 beats per minute.

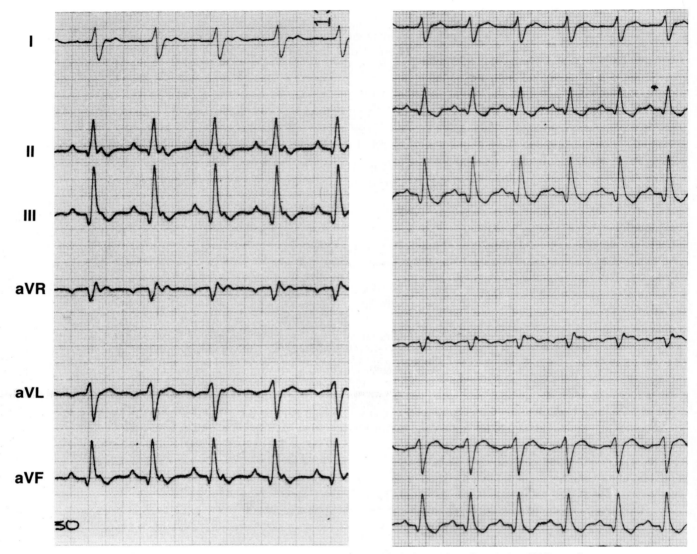

Figure 8–2. (*Left panel*) Atrial tachycardia with 2:1 AV block due to digitalis toxicity. (*Right panel*) Same patient during sinus rhythm. In the *left panel*, note the typical features of digitalis-induced atrial tachycardia: (1) superior/inferior atrial activation, indicating an origin high in the right atrium; (2) ventriculophasic PP intervals during 2:1 AV block (i.e., the PP interval embracing the R wave is shorter than the PP without an R).

2. There is usually 2:1 AV block or AV Wenckebach.
3. P axis is usually directed inferiorly (P wave positive in leads II, III, and aVF).
4. Ventriculophasic PP intervals are often present.

    When digitalis is discontinued, transient 1:1 conduction may appear before the rhythm converts to sinus rhythm. Because the focus is frequently high in the right atrium close to the sinus node, the P waves of this tachycardia closely resemble sinus P waves.

Ventriculophasic PP Intervals

Often in atrial tachycardia due to digitalis toxicity there is ventriculophasic behavior of PP intervals (i.e., the PP interval embracing the R wave is shorter than the PP interval without an R wave). The fact that the P wave following the QRS is somewhat premature may cause a misdiagnosis of bigeminal nonconducted premature atrial complexes by the uninformed. The mechanism of ventriculophasic changes in PP intervals is the same as that seen in complete heart block (i.e., peak vagal activity occurs just after the aortic pressure wave reaches the baroreceptors of the carotid body). This causes the next atrial cycle (without a QRS complex) to lengthen.[10-12]

Figure 8–2 shows in the left panel an atrial tachycardia with 2:1 AV block in a patient taking digitalis. Note that the distance between the P waves on either side of the QRS is shorter than that between the P waves without the QRS (ventriculophasic PP intervals). Other features of digitalis toxicity in this patient are the polarity of the P waves (similar to sinus P waves, i.e., upright in leads II, III, and aVF) and the atrial rate.

AV JUNCTIONAL TACHYCARDIA

The ECG features of AV junctional tachycardia due to digitalis toxicity are:

1. Rate: 70 to 140 per minute
2. Nonparoxysmal
3. Rate increase with exercise
4. Carotid sinus massage has no effect or there may be nodoventricular block.
5. AV dissociation (usually)

Because of its gradual onset, this tachycardia is called "nonparoxysmal."[13] Its rate rarely exceeds 140 per minute, and it begins to show itself when its rate is faster than that of the sinus rhythm, usually at about 70 per minute. There is AV dissociation, and the term "accelerated AV junctional rhythm" is generally applied (Fig. 8–3). When the rate exceeds 100 per minute it is the same mechanism, although it now may be called "AV junctional tachycardia." The difficulty with this change in terms is that a different mechanism is suggested, although actually triggered activity in the AV junction is responsible for both. The tachycardia is usually associated with AV dissociation because of the blocking effect of digitalis on anterograde and retrograde conduction in the AV node.

ATRIAL FIBRILLATION

When AV junctional tachycardia occurs in atrial fibrillation, it is initially recognized because of a more regular ventricular rhythm than would be expected during atrial fibrillation. This may later become completely regular if digitalis is not discontinued. Figure 8–4 is an example of regularization of the ventricular rhythm during atrial fibrillation. The atria are fibrillating and the ventricles are now under the control of an accelerated AV junctional

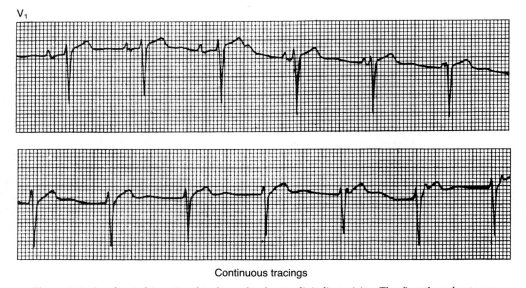

Continuous tracings

Figure 8–3. Accelerated junctional tachycardia due to digitalis toxicity. The first three beats are sinus impulses that are conducted to the ventricles. When the sinus rate slows, the junctional rhythm takes over.

focus. Exit block from a junctional focus is also possible. In such a case there would be group beating, such as is seen during atrial fibrillation in Figure 8–5. It is very important to be aware of this mechanism and to rule it out when evaluating a patient with atrial fibrillation, because at first glance the rhythm appears appropriately irregular. The tracing in Figure 8–6 shows atrial fibrillation with complete AV block and AV junctional escape pacemaker.

ATRIAL FLUTTER

The emergence of junctional tachycardia due to digitalis toxicity in atrial flutter is even more subtle than in atrial fibrillation, and the toxicity may go on for days or even weeks without being recognized on the ECG.

In uncomplicated atrial flutter there is usually 2:1 AV conduction or Wenckebach conduction. When the conduction ratio is constant (e.g., 2:1 or 4:1) the relationship between the flutter wave and the R wave is identical every time. Sometimes during atrial flutter there is 2:1 conduction in the upper AV node and Wenckebach conduction in the lower AV node, resulting in the typical group beating of Wenckebach periods, and the flutter-QRS relationship is identical every other time for both sets of beats.

In atrial flutter with AV block and/or an accelerated idiojunctional rhythm or junctional tachycardia due to digitalis toxicity, the ventricular rhythm is regular and the flutter-QRS relationship varies (Fig. 8–7).

Other causes of accelerated junctional rhythm and junctional tachycardia besides digitalis are ischemia, myocarditis, and electrolyte disturbances; they may also occur following open heart surgery.

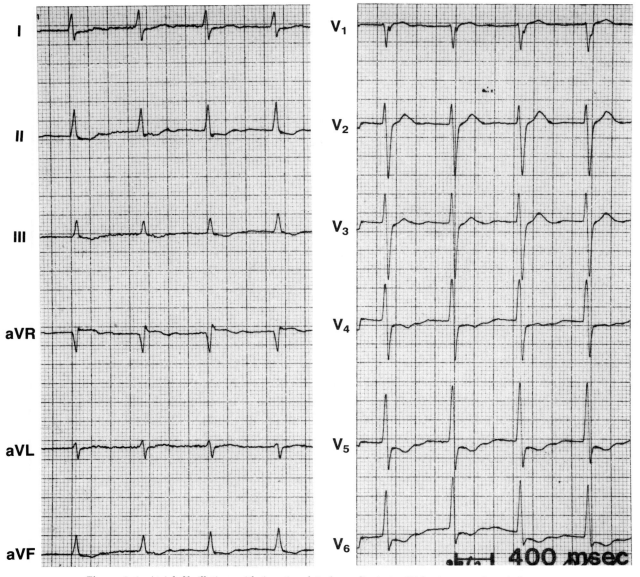

Figure 8–4. Atrial fibrillation with junctional tachycardia (rate: 95 beats per minute) due to digitalis toxicity. Note the absolute regularity of the rhythm.

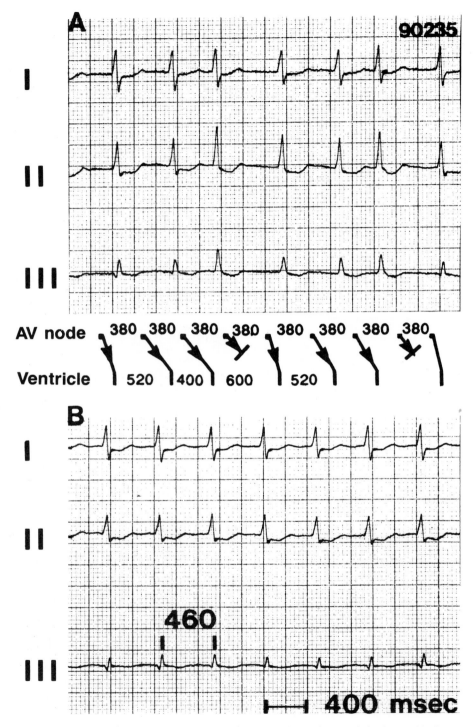

Figure 8–5. Atrial fibrillation and junctional tachycardia with Wenckebach exit block. In *panel A*, note the group beating. The mechanism is explained in the diagram. *Panel B*, recorded 1 day later, shows junctional tachycardia at a slower rate, allowing 1:1 conduction from the focus to the ventricle.

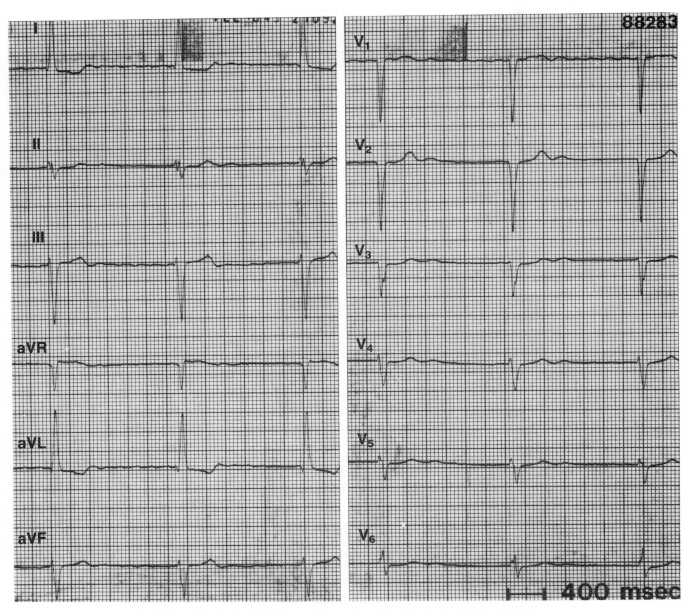

Figure 8–6. Atrial fibrillation with complete AV block due to digitalis toxicity.

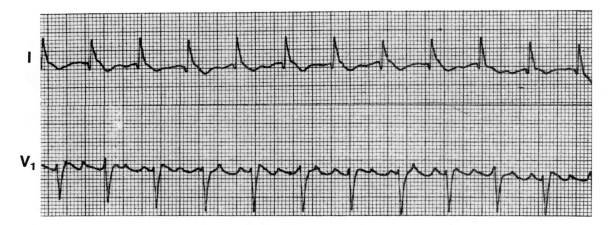

Figure 8–7. Atrial flutter with AV dissociation due to junctional tachycardia secondary to digitalis toxicity. Tracing is postoperative. The junctional rate is 112 beats per minute. (Courtesy of William P. Nelson, M.D.)

FASCICULAR VENTRICULAR TACHYCARDIA

The ECG features of fascicular ventricular tachycardia are:

1. Rate: 90 to 160 per minute
2. RBBB shape (usually)
3. QRS 0.12 to 0.14 sec
4. Axis deviation (right or left)

One of the ventricular ectopic rhythms common to digitalis toxicity is fascicular ventricular tachycardia, in which the location of impulse formation is in one of the bundle branches, commonly the anterior or posterior fascicle of the left bundle branch. Another feature of such a tachycardia, in addition to the ones listed above, is that changes may occur in QRS configuration due to competition between Purkinje fibers for the pacing role. As with the other digitalis dysrhythmias, its emergence is promoted by the shortening of the cycle lengths of preceding beats and by catecholamines. Short cycle lengths and increased sympathetic tone cause an otherwise "dormant" delayed afterdepolarization to reach threshold potential and produce triggered activity. Figure 8–8 is an example of atrial fibrillation with fascicular ventricular tachycardia due to digitalis toxicity. Note the relatively narrow QRS, the RBBB pattern in lead V_1, and right axis deviation. In Figure 8–9 there are a double tachycardia, atrial tachycardia, and fascicular ventricular tachycardia.

Right Bundle Branch Block Pattern

The RBBB pattern in lead V_1 and the QRS width of less than 0.14 sec are due to a focus within the left bundle branch. In such a case, the left ventricle would be activated before the right, just as it is when there is RBBB.

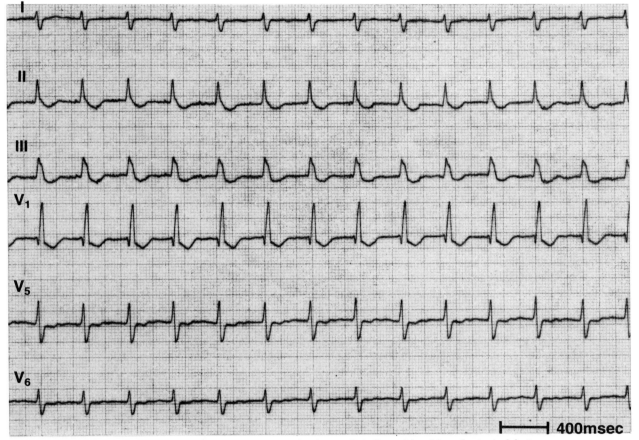

Figure 8–8. Fascicular ventricular tachycardia due to digitalis toxicity. Note the typical features of this arrhythmia: QRS < 0.14 second, RBBB pattern, and right axis deviation, indicating an origin of the arrhythmia in the left anterior fascicle.

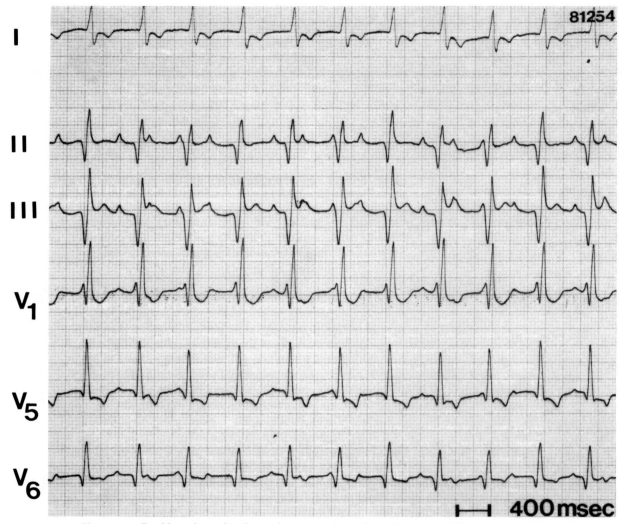

Figure 8–9. Double tachycardia: Fascicular ventricular tachycardia (rate 110 beats per minute) and atrial tachycardia (rate 180 beats per minute) due to digitalis toxicity. Note the typical RBBB pattern and P wave morphology (similar to sinus P waves). The right axis deviation of the ventricular tachycardia indicates an origin of this arrhythmia in the left anterior fascicle.

QRS Duration

The QRS duration is not as broad as would be expected in ventricular tachycardia because the impulse formation in fascicular ventricular tachycardia occurs within the conduction system, and therefore it gains access to the remainder of the conduction system rapidly, not being dependent on ventricular myocardium.

Axis Deviation

Axis deviation is a typical finding in fascicular ventricular tachycardia; whether it is right or left depends on the site of origin in the fascicle (anterior or posterior) of the left bundle branch. When there is right axis deviation, the focus is in the anterior (superior) fascicle. When the axis deviation is left, there is a posterior (inferior) fascicular focus.

BIDIRECTIONAL VENTRICULAR TACHYCARDIA

The ECG features of bidirectional ventricular tachycardia are:

1. Rate: 90 to 160 per minute
2. RBBB shape
3. QRS 0.12 to 0.14 sec
4. Alternating axis deviation (right/left)

Bidirectional ventricular tachycardia has long been recognized clinically as one of the signs of severe digitalis toxicity. The ECG resembles that in fascicular ventricular tachycardia except that an alternating pattern of RBBB and left axis deviation and RBBB and right axis deviation is present, leading to the "bidirectional" look of the tachycardia in the limb leads (Fig. 8–10). The mechanism of bidirectional ventricular tachycardia is thought to be alternating impulse formation in the left anterior and left posterior fascicles.

VENTRICULAR BIGEMINY

Figure 8–11 is an example of ventricular bigeminy due to digitalis toxicity. Although ventricular bigeminy may occur in digitalis toxicity, its most common cause is coronary artery disease. In a series of 100 patients with ventricular bigeminy, 79 percent were not taking digitalis but had coronary artery disease.[10]

Because Purkinje fibers compete for the pacing role, if a long enough tracing is taken, you may note that the ventricular ectopic beats may have different configurations even though the coupling interval is fixed.[10]

SINUS BRADYCARDIA AND SINOATRIAL BLOCK

Digitalis suppresses phase 4 depolarization and causes conduction problems in the SA region. Thus, sinus bradycardia, sinus arrest, and SA Wenckebach may result from digitalis toxicity. SA Wenckebach is diagnosed when there

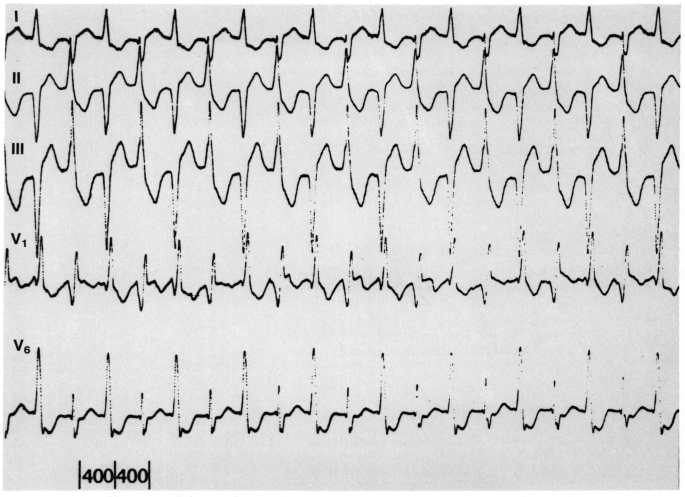

Figure 8–10. Bidirectional ventricular tachycardia due to digitalis toxicity. Note the typical features: RBBB pattern, relatively narrow QRS (0.12 sec), and alternating left and right axis deviation, indicating alternating impulse formation in the left posterior and anterior fascicles.

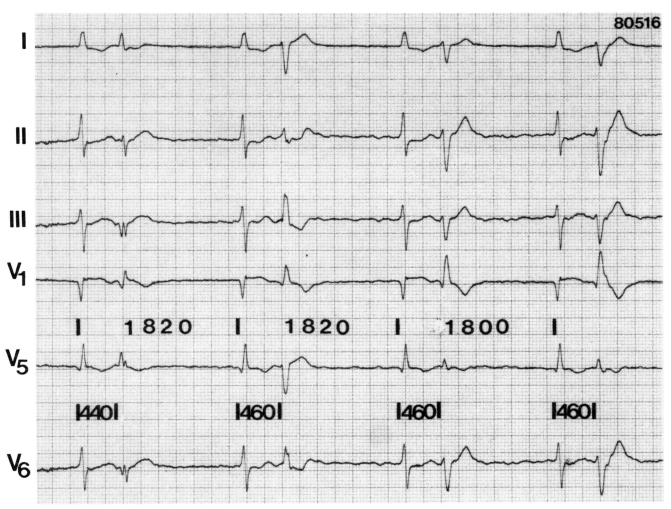

Figure 8–11. Ventricular bigeminy due to digitalis toxicity. Note that the patient has atrial fibrillation with high-degree AV block. Note also that in spite of few or no changes in coupling interval, the ventricular premature beats differ in configuration because of a different site of origin in the Purkinje system of the left ventricle.

is group beating of the P waves with progressive shortening of the PP interval before the blocked beat. The ECG features of SA Wenckebach are illustrated in Figure 8–12. However, in digitalis toxicity the SA Wenckebach or complete SA block (see Fig. 5–5) is frequently combined with AV Wenckebach and/or junctional tachycardia or fascicular ventricular tachycardia, and the combination can present a very challenging and complicated tracing. A systematic approach to the ECG is imperative and is covered in this chapter.

ATRIOVENTRICULAR NODAL WENCKEBACH

AV nodal Wenckebach conduction can be found in digitalis toxicity. Digitalis lengthens the refractory period of AV nodal tissue, leading to progressive PR prolongation before a P wave fails to be conducted to the ventricles.

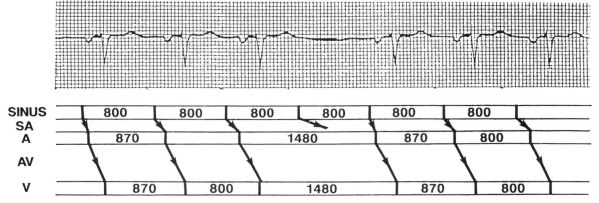

Figure 8–12. SA Wenckebach. The sinus impulse is discharging at regular intervals (800 msec). There is Wenckebach conduction from the sinus node to the atrium. The progressively lengthening SA conduction times eventually culminate in a nonconducted sinus impulse (no P wave). Because the greatest increment in conduction is between the first and second P waves, the typical features of Wenckebach conduction can be seen (i.e., group beating, shortening PP intervals, and pauses that are less than twice the shortest cycle).

NON-ECG SIGNS OF DIGITALIS TOXICITY

Many factors determine whether a given blood level of digitalis is actually toxic. Thus, serum concentrations should not be used as the basis for evaluating toxicity. The ECG and symptoms should be of more value to the clinician in making these decisions.

Take a history and ask the patient and family specific questions regarding medication being taken, noticeable changes in color vision, and changes in behavior, such as lack of energy or memory (pseudodementia). Usually, neither the patient nor the family members will volunteer these complaints, and they must be prompted with questions regarding a change in the clearness of the colors on television, clearness of the print when reading the newspaper, loss of interest in surroundings, and so forth.

Other noncardiac signs and symptoms of digitalis intoxication are gastrointestinal (nausea, vomiting, diarrhea, abdominal pain, anorexia); visual (ptosis), neurologic and muscular (fatigue, weakness), hallucinations, nightmares, restlessness, insomnia, listlessness, and so forth.

TREATMENT OF DIGITALIS DYSRHYTHMIAS

1. Discontinue the drug.
2. Bedrest (no sympathetic stimulation)
3. Correct electrolyte abnormalities.
4. Active treatment of a rapid ventricular rhythm depends upon the site of origin of the arrhythmia and its hemodynamic consequences.
5. If the arrhythmia is ventricular in origin, especially when a bidirectional tachycardia is present, give phenytoin or digitalis antibodies.

6. A ventricular pacing lead should be inserted if phenytoin is used because the drug may not only suppress the arrhythmia, thereby exposing high-degree block, but it may also prevent escape rhythms from occurring because digitalis depresses phase 4 depolarization in His-Purkinje cells.

7. Ventricular pacing is indicated when digitalis-induced bradycardia by SA block and/or AV block lead to hemodynamic deterioration.

DANGERS OF PACING AND CAROTID SINUS MASSAGE

- Rapid pacing in a patient with an arrhythmia based upon delayed after-depolarization may cause acceleration of the arrhythmia.
- Sudden cessation of pacing may cause asystole because of failure of escape beats due to the depressed phase 4 depolarization in His-Purkinje cells.
- In patients with digitalis intoxication, carotid sinus massage has been reported to result in worsening of the arrhythmias and induction of ventricular fibrillation.

A SYSTEMATIC EVALUATION OF PATIENTS TAKING DIGITALIS

The arrhythmias in the setting of digitalis toxicity may be complex because there may be more than one focus of abnormal impulse formation (e.g., atrial tachycardia in combination with junctional or fascicular ventricular tachycardia). There may also be a combination of blocks such as AV nodal and SA nodal. Thus, the ECG is approached very systematically after the history is taken. Table 8–2 and the points listed below provide a guide for evaluating the ECG of patients who are taking digitalis.

1. Talk to your patient, inquiring about the dose of digitalis, additional medication, and complaints such as visual and gastrointestinal symptoms.

2. Talk to the patient's family, inquiring about the patient's complaints and personality changes.

3. Before looking at the ECG, review what abnormalities can be encountered as dysrhythmic expressions of digitalis toxicity.

4. Evaluate the ECG systematically (Table 8–2), starting at the top of the heart (SA nodal function? atrial tachycardia?) and then down through the AV node (AV block? junctional tachycardia?), into the His-Purkinje system (fascicular ventricular tachycardia? bidirectional ventricular tachycardia? ventricular bigeminy?). Such an approach will help to reveal the double tachycardias such as atrial tachycardia and fascicular ventricular tachycardia, or the atrial tachycardia that is combined with AV conduction abnormalities.

5. When the patient with atrial fibrillation is taking digitalis, although the rate slows, the rhythm should remain totally irregular. Regularization indicates either a junctional or ventricular rhythm, which can be rapid (70–140 beats per minute) or slow, as in complete AV block. Group

Table 8–2. **Systematic Evaluation of the ECG for Digitalis Toxicity**

P Wave Regularity, Rate, and Polarity
If irregular, SA block?
If rate >120 beats/min, evaluate polarity in leads II and aVF
Atrial tachycardia?

AV Conduction
Signs of AV Wenckebach?
Signs of complete AV block?

AV Junctional Rhythm
Are all QRS complexes conducted?
If not, what is the rate of the AV junctional focus?
Is tachycardia paroxysmal or nonparoxysmal?
If nonparoxysmal and the rate is 70–130 beats/min—digitalis-toxic AV junctional tachycardia

Fascicular Ventricular Tachycardia
Are the ventricular complexes conducted from the atrium?
If not, what is the rate?
If 90–160 beats/min, suspect fascicular ventricular tachycardia
What is the morphology in lead V_1?
If RBBB, what is the axis?
If abnormal—fascicular ventricular tachycardia

Atrial Fibrillation
Is the rhythm intermittently or completely regular?
What is the QRS morphology in lead V_1?
- If RBBB, suspect fascicular ventricular tachycardia due to digitalis toxicity
- If normal, suspect a junctional rhythm due to junctional tachycardia and/or AV block secondary to digitalis toxicity

Atrial Flutter
Does the flutter–R wave relationship have a pattern? (Fixed? Alternative?)
If not, is the ventricular rhythm regular?
If so—AV dissociation; assess ventricular rate and QRS morphology
- If ventricular rate <60 beats/min—atrial flutter with complete AV block
- If QRS is normal and rate 70–140 beats/min—atrial flutter with AV dissociation and AV junctional tachycardia due to digitalis toxicity
- If RBBB and rate 90–160 beats/min—atrial flutter, AV dissociation, and fascicular ventricular tachycardia due to digitalis toxicity

beating in atrial fibrillation with a narrow QRS suggests junctional tachycardia with Wenckebach exit block.

6. If there is atrial flutter, the flutter–R wave relationship should be constant or vary in a repetitive fashion as it would with Wenckebach conduction; this is not the case when digitalis toxicity causes complete AV block and accelerated AV junctional impulse formation. The ECG then shows varying flutter–R wave relationships with a regular ventricular rhythm.

SUMMARY

The mortality associated with digitalis toxicity often goes unrecognized because the poisoning process is slow and the patient is being treated for heart problems, which are ultimately blamed for his or her demise. Toxicity is diagnosed because of subjective and ECG symptoms, digitalis blood level being unreliable as a sole indicator. Digitalis causes SA and AV conduction problems. The foci for tachycardia can be located in the atrium, AV junction, and the fascicles of the bundle branches.

These arrhythmias have diagnostic features. In atrial tachycardia the P waves are usually positive in leads II, III, and aVF; the rate is between 130 and 250 beats per minute; there are often ventriculophasic behavior of the PP intervals and 2:1 AV block. In junctional tachycardia there is usually retrograde block (AV dissociation), the rate is between 70 and 140 beats per minute, and the rhythm begins gradually (nonparoxysmal). In fascicular ventricular tachycardia the rate is between 90 and 160 beats per minute; the QRS shows right bundle branch block configuration, and it measures between 0.12 and 0.14 sec.

Emergency management consists of discontinuing the digitalis, bedrest, and correction of electrolyte abnormalities. The use of phenytoin and ventricular pacing or digitalis antibodies depends upon the site of origin and hemodynamic consequences of the arrhythmia.

References

1. Dreifus, L.S., McKnight, E.H., Katz, M., et al.: Digitalis intolerance. Geriatrics 18:494–502, 1963.
2. Katz, A.M.: Effects of digitalis on cell biochemistry: Sodium pump inhibition. J. Am. Coll. Cardiol. 5:16A, 1985.
3. Rosen, M.R.: The relationship of delayed afterdepolarizations to arrhythmias in the intact heart. PACE 6:1151, 1983.
4. Gadsby, D.C., and Wit, A.L.: Normal and abnormal electrical activity in cardiac cells. In: Mandel W.J.: Cardiac Arrhythmias. Philadelphia, 1987, Lippincott, pp. 53–80.
5. Gorgels, A.P.M., Vos, M.A., Brugada, P., et al.: The clinical relevance of abnormal automaticity and triggered activity. In Brugada, P., and Wellens, H.J.J.: Cardiac Arrhythmias: Where To Go From Here? Mount Kisco, NY, 1987, Futura, pp. 147–169.
6. Wellens, H.J.J.: The electrocardiogram in digitalis intoxication. In Yu, P.N., and Goodwin, J.F. (eds.): Progress in Cardiology, Vol. 5. Philadelphia, 1976, Lea & Febiger, pp. 271–290.
7. Marcus, F.I.: Pharmacokinetic interactions between digoxin and other drugs. J. Am. Coll. Cardiol. 5:82A–90A, 1985.
8. Klein, H.O., Lang, R., Weiss, E., et al.: The influence of verapamil on serum digoxin concentration. Circulation 65:998–1003, 1982.
9. Rosen, M.R., Fisch, C., Hoffman, B.F., et al.: Can accelerated atrioventricular junctional escape rhythms be explained by delayed afterdepolarizations? Am. J. Cardiol. 45:1272–1284, 1980.
10. Vanagt, E.J., and Wellens, H.J.J.: The electrocardiogram in digitalis intoxication. In Wellens, H.J.J., and Kulbertus, H.E. (eds.): What's New in Electrocardiography? The Hague, 1981, Martinus Nijhoff, pp. 315–343.
11. Roth, I.R., and Kish, B.: Mechanisms of irregular sinus rhythm in auriculoventricular heart block. Am. Heart J. 36:257–276, 1948.
12. Rosenbaum, M.B., and Lepeschkin, E.: Effects of ventricular systole on auricular rhythm in auriculo-ventricular block. Circulation 11:240–261, 1955.
13. Pick, A., and Dominguez, P.: Nonparoxysmal A-V nodal tachycardia. Circulation 16:1022–1032, 1957.

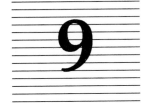

C H A P T E R

9

Other Drug-Induced Emergencies

EMERGENCY TREATMENT

TORSADE DE POINTES

1. Stop the offending drug.
2. Continue ECG monitoring.
3. Give magnesium as MgCl or $MgSO_4$ 1 to 2 gm IV bolus over 5 minutes; infusion: 1 to 2 gm per hour for 4 to 6 hours.
4. If IV magnesium is unsuccessful, increase heart rate with isoproterenol or by pacing.

SUSTAINED (INCESSANT) MONOMORPHIC VENTRICULAR TACHYCARDIA

1. Stop the offending drug.
2. In case of hemodynamic compromise, give inotropic support with isoproterenol or epinephrine. This will also counteract slowing in conduction velocity induced by class IA or class IC drugs.
3. If ventricular tachycardia persists and is poorly tolerated, pace the atrium at the rate of the ventricular tachycardia. Use an AV interval that will provide maximal contribution of atrial contraction to ventricular filling.

DRUG-INDUCED BRADYCARDIA

1. Stop the offending drug.
2. Give atropine or start temporary transvenous pacing in case of (a) Adams-Stokes attacks, (b) a low ventricular rate leading to hypotension, and/or (c) bradycardia-dependent ventricular arrhythmias.

INTRODUCTION

Antiarrhythmic drugs may worsen the cardiac rhythm in 10 percent to 15 percent of patients suffering from an arrhythmia. Therefore, when a patient receives antiarrhythmic drug therapy, the situation may worsen instead of improve. This may vary from (1) a marked increase in ectopic atrial or

MECHANISM OF ARRHYTHMIAS

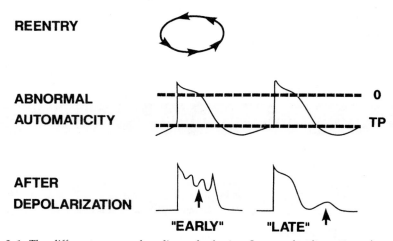

Figure 9–1. The different causes of cardiac arrhythmias. See text for discussion of reentry and arrhythmias based on "early" or "late" afterdepolarizations. The role of abnormal automaticity in drug-induced arrhythmias is not clear at the present time.

ventricular activity or (2) a change from a nonsustained to a sustained tachycardia, to (3) the development of torsade de pointes or (4) high-degree sinoatrial (SA) or atrioventricular (AV) block.

MECHANISMS

Two mechanisms are thought to be responsible for the proarrhythmic effect of antiarrhythmic drugs: (1) re-entry and (2) triggered activity, which may be caused by either delayed or early afterdepolarizations (Fig. 9–1). Re-entry may be facilitated because the drug slows conduction without sufficient prolongation of the refractory period in the reentry circuit. Early afterdepolarizations may occur following the administration of drugs that prolong the refractory period (class IA and class III drugs). Delayed afterdepolarizations do occur in digitalis intoxication (see Chapter 8).

REENTRY

During reentry, an impulse circulates in a circuit composed of cardiac fibers somewhere in the heart. Such a mechanism requires (1) an initiating stimulus, which is conducted only one way within the circuit; (2) slow conduction through at least one portion of the circuit; and (3) a circuit long enough to allow recovery of the tissue ahead of the circulating impulse (Fig. 9–2).

Thus, antiarrhythmic drugs (such as class IC drugs encainide and flecainide) that slow conduction without lengthening the refractory period may facilitate the occurrence and perpetuation of a reentry mechanism.

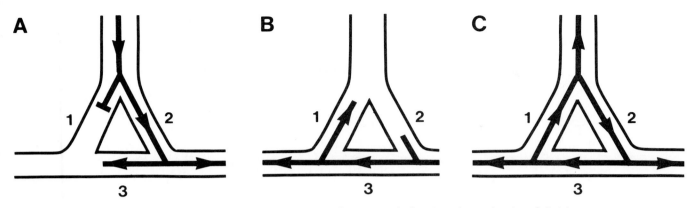

Figure 9–2. Mechanism of reentry. *Panel A* shows arrival of an impulse at the site of division into two pathways. Because of differences in the duration of the refractory periods of the two pathways, the impulse is blocked in one pathway and not the other (pathway 1 has the longer refractory period). *Panel B* shows how the impulse emerging from pathway 2 can reenter pathway 1 (via 3). If the proximal portion of pathway 1 has recovered, the impulse is able to return to the site of origin. *Panel C*: If this mechanism perpetuates, a regular tachycardia results due to reentry.

TRIGGERED ACTIVITY

Triggered activity, apart from being based upon delayed afterdepolarizations (Chapter 8), may be caused by early afterdepolarizations.

Early afterdepolarizations are oscillations in the transmembrane potential that occur before the completion of phase 3 repolarization (Fig. 9–1). If such oscillations reach threshold potential, triggered activity results (tachycardia). The occurrence of arrhythmias based upon early afterdepolarizations is favored by a slow heart rate and prolonged phase 2 and phase 3 of the membrane action potential.

Both class IA drugs, such as quinidine, procainamide, and disopyramide, and class III drugs, which include sotalol and amiodarone, lengthen the membrane action potential duration, prolong the QT interval, and may therefore promote the occurrence of early afterdepolarizations and ventricular arrhythmias. These arrhythmias may have a polymorphic form and have been named "torsade de pointes." They usually occur early (i.e., a few hours to a few days after the administration of the class IA or class III drugs), suggesting that this is not a toxic but an idiosyncratic reaction to the drug. Their occurrence is promoted by hypokalemia and hypomagnesemia.

TORSADE DE POINTES

Torsade de pointes is a type of polymorphic ventricular tachycardia associated with marked QT prolongation.[1] It may occur after administration of class IA and class III antiarrhythmic drugs. The tachycardia is paroxysmal and may result in ventricular fibrillation and sudden death. Its onset is promoted by a slow basic rhythm and frequently follows a pause induced

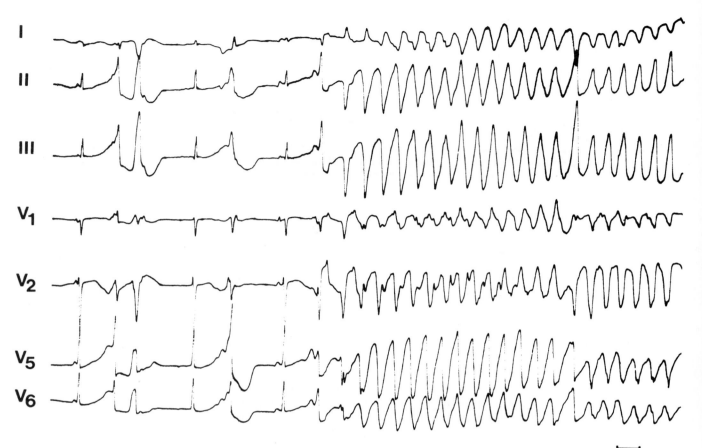

400 msec

Figure 9–3. Torsade de pointes. Note (1) the prolonged QT interval; (2) the long–short cycles preceding the onset of the tachycardia; and (3) the typical oscillating morphology of the ventricular complexes.

by a premature ventricular contraction (PVC) (Fig. 9–3). The tachycardia is characterized by polymorphic QRS complexes.

ECG DIAGNOSIS

1. Lengthening of the QT interval
2. Prominent U wave of the conducted sinus beats
3. A long–short cycle frequently initiates the tachycardia (Fig. 9–3).
4. Polymorphic oscillations in the QRS height during the tachycardia
5. The tachycardia rate varies from 200 to 400 beats per minute.

WARNING SIGNS

Progressive lengthening of the QT interval and the development of a prominent U wave are important warning signs. The degree of QT prolon-

OTHER DRUG-INDUCED EMERGENCIES

gation that predicts torsade de pointes is not known. In quinidine-induced torsade de pointes the QT intervals may exceed 0.60 sec. Figure 9–4 illustrates the long QT interval and U wave of a patient taking sotalol.

EMERGENCY TREATMENT

Class IA drug-induced torsade de pointes and that induced by sotalol (a class III drug) usually appear early after the drug treatment has been initiated and the patient is still in the hospital. In this setting, detection and treatment should be early and relatively easy. The following measures are taken for the treatment of torsade de pointes:

1. Continuous monitoring
2. Discontinuation of the offending drug
3. Correction of electrolyte abnormalities with potassium and magnesium
4. Intravenous magnesium is suggested even in normomagnesemia.[2, 3] Give MgCl or $MgSO_4$ 1 to 2 gm IV bolus over 5 minutes; infusion: 1 to 2 gm

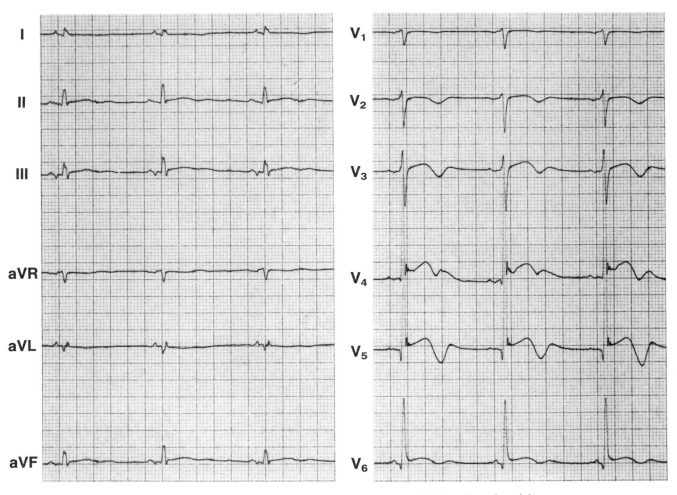

Figure 9–4. Prolonged QT interval and U wave due to administration of sotalol.

per hour for 4 to 6 hours. MgCl is preferred to $MgSO_4$ because sulfate binds calcium and chloride does not.

5. If IV magnesium is unsuccessful, an increase in basic heart rate with isoproterenol or by ventricular pacing may be necessary.

CLASS IC DRUG-RELATED EMERGENCIES

Class IC drugs include flecainide, encainide, indecainide, recainam, and propafenone. The emergence of a sustained ventricular tachycardia after starting such a drug or after an increase in drug dose suggests an adverse drug effect. The drug dose does not have to be toxic but merely large enough to slow conduction velocity suffiently to facilitate circulation of the impulse within the reentry circuit. In contrast to the occurrence of torsade de pointes, which is promoted by a slow heart rate, induction of ventricular tachycardia by a class IC drug is promoted by a fast heart rate (Fig. 9–5). This is because slowing in conduction velocity after the administration of class IC drugs becomes more marked when the heart rate is increased.

CHARACTERISTICS

The ventricular tachycardia caused by class IC drugs has the following clinical signs:

1. Spontaneous onset after starting the drug or increasing the dose
2. Sustained or persistent nature
3. The ventricular tachycardia shows very wide QRS complexes because of slowing in conduction velocity of the circulating impulse by the class IC drug. Ventricular tachycardia can frequently not be terminated by cardioversion or programmed ventricular stimulation or it resumes after only one or two sinus beats.

EMERGENCY TREATMENT

1. Stop the offending drug.
2. In case of hemodynamic compromise, give inotropic support with isoproterenol or epinephrine. This will also counteract slowing in conduction velocity induced by class IA or class IC drugs.
3. In case of persistence of ventricular tachycardia, pace the atrium at the rate of the ventricular tachycardia using an AV interval that allows for maximal contribution of atrial contraction to the ventricular filling.

DRUG-INDUCED BRADYCARDIA

As shown in Table 9–1, several drugs may produce bradycardia by creating sinus bradycardia, SA block, AV nodal block, or subnodal block.

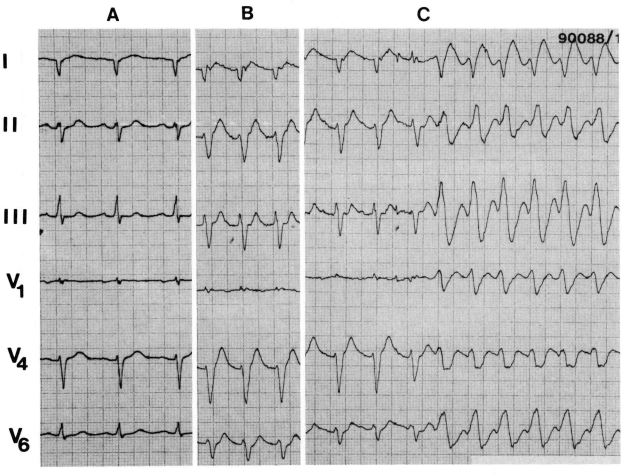

Figure 9–5. Initiation of a sustained ventricular tachycardia during exercise testing in a patient receiving a class IC agent. *Panel A*: Before exercise. The heart rate is 80 beats per minute and the QRS width measures 100 msec. *Panel B*: During exercise. The heart rate is 130 beats per minute, QRS width is 160 msec, and there is left axis deviation. *Panel C*: Shortly thereafter a ventricular tachycardia begins with a rate of 150 beats per minute.

Sinus bradycardia may be caused by beta-blocking agents like propranolol and metoprolol.

SA block may be the result of treatment with class IA drugs (quinidine, procainamide, disopyramide), class IC drugs (encainide, flecainide, propafenone), beta-blocking agents, class III drugs (sotalol, amiodarone), and digitalis.

AV nodal block may occur after the administration of beta-blocking agents, class III drugs, calcium antagonists (verapamil, diltiazem), and digitalis.

Sub–AV nodal (His–Purkinje) block may be induced by class IA drugs, class IB drugs (mexiletine, tocainide), class IC drugs, and class III drugs.

Table 9–1. **Possible Sites of Block in Relation to Different Types (Classes) of Antiarrhythmic Drugs**

Class	Site of Block		
	Sinoatrial	*AV Nodal*	*His-Bundle Branches*
IA quinidine procainamide disopyramide ajmaline	+	−	+
IB tocainide mexiletine	−	−	+
IC encainide flecainide propafenone	+	+	+
II beta-blocking drugs	+	+	−
III amiodarone sotalol	+	+	+
IV verapamil diltiazem	−	+	−
Digitalis	+	+	−

EMERGENCY TREATMENT

1. Stop the offending drug.
2. Give atropine or start temporary tranvenous pacing in case of (a) Adams-Stokes attacks, (b) a low ventricular rate leading to hypotension and/or congestive failure, or (c) bradycardia-dependent ventricular arrhythmias.

SUMMARY

Antiarrhythmic drugs may induce tachycardia or block, worsening the patient's arrhythmias. This possibility should always be suspected when a patient reports worsening of his or her condition after the start of the antiarrhythmic drug therapy.

References

1. Dessertenne, F.: Complexes électrique ventriculaire à phase lente prolongée. Semin. Hosp. Paris 43:539–547, 1967.
2. Iseri, L.T., Chung, P., and Tobis, J.: Magnesium therapy for intractable ventricular tachyarrhythmias in normomagnesemic patients. West. J. Med. 138:823–828, 1983.
3. Etienne, Y., Blanc, J.J., Songy, B., et al.: Antiarrhythmic effects of intravenous magnesium sulfate in torsade de pointes. (Apropos of 6 cases.) Arch. Malad. Coeur Vais. 79(3):362–367, 1986.

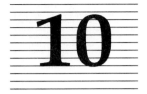

CHAPTER

10

Potassium-Related Emergencies

EMERGENCY APPROACH TO HYPO- AND HYPERKALEMIA

ECG RECOGNITION OF SEVERE OR PROGRESSIVE HYPERKALEMIA

- Broad QRS
- Slow heart rate
- Usually left axis deviation
- Loss of P wave
- Loss of ST segment (continuous with S wave)
- Tall tented T wave
- QTc interval normal or shortened

TREATMENT

1. Calcium gluconate (10 percent) 10 to 30 ml IV infusion over 1 to 5 minutes with constant ECG monitoring
2. Hypertonic glucose solution (10 percent) 200 to 500 ml in 30 minutes, and 500 to 1000 ml over the next several hours
3. Sodium bicarbonate (2 to 3 ampuls) may be added to 1 liter of 5 percent dextrose in 0.9 percent saline.
4. Cation exchange resins (sodium polystyrene sulfonate) by retention enema; this may be repeated until potassium levels are within safe limits. Oral doses of 20 gm are given 3 or 4 times a day together with 20 ml of 70 percent sorbitol solution.
5. If renal failure: hemodialysis or peritoneal dialysis along with one of the treatments above

ECG RECOGNITION OF SEVERE HYPOKALEMIA (SERUM LEVEL OF LESS THAN 2.5 mEq/L)

- ST depression
- Decrease in T wave amplitude
- Increase in U wave amplitude

> **TREATMENT**
> 1. Potassium chloride IV not to exceed 40 mEq/L at an infusion rate not to exceed 20 mEq/hour (approximately 200 to 250 mEq/day)
> 2. Oral potassium chloride

POTASSIUM

The potassium ion plays a key role in the normal function of the cells of the human body.[1] In the heart, specific levels of intra- and extracellular potassium are essential for normal impulse generation and conduction.

Potassium is excreted by the body in the urine, feces, and perspiration. Diuretics, vomiting, perspiration, and diarrhea can rapidly deplete the body of this vital ion (hypokalemia). Conversely, anuria can cause a potassium buildup (hyperkalemia). Both conditions may produce serious arrhythmias and even death.

The potassium gradient across the cell membrane, along with the intracellular negativity generated by the sodium pump, determines the resting membrane potential and thus conduction velocity and help to confine pacing activity to the sinus node. In the resting state, approximately 30 times as much potassium is within a cell as is in the extracellular fluid. A normal gradient and normal sodium-potassium pump activity create a resting membrane potential of -90 mV, which in turn permits rapid depolarization (phase 0 of the membrane potential), leading to optimal stimulation of neighboring cells.

HYPERKALEMIA

MECHANISM

An increase in extracellular potassium decreases the gradient of potassium across the cell membrane, thereby reducing the resting membrane potential. This in turn reduces the height and steepness of phase 0 of the action potential and slows conduction. Furthermore, the velocity of phase 3 (terminal repolarization) is accelerated and the action potential duration shortens. This results in a typical ECG picture when the serum potassium level exceeds 5.5 mEq/L.

ECG CHANGES IN PROGRESSIVE HYPERKALEMIA

Figure 10–1 is a schematic representation of the ECG changes as the serum concentration passes from normal to 8 mEq/L.[2, 3]

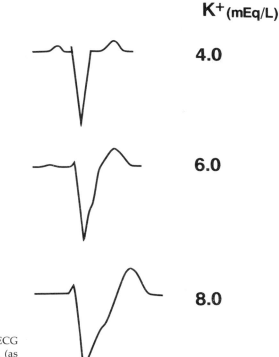

K^+(mEq/L)

4.0

6.0

8.0

Figure 10–1. A representation of the ECG changes in progressive hyperkalemia (as seen in lead V_1).

MILD HYPERKALEMIA (BELOW 6.0 mEq/L)

Because of slowing in conduction, the P wave widens with a loss in height, the PR interval is prolonged, and the QRS complex widens. The T wave becomes tall and tented without prolongation of the QTc.

SEVERE HYPERKALEMIA (ABOVE 6.0 mEq/L)

Above 6.0 mEq/L, there is further widening of the QRS complex, primarily the second portion of the QRS complex, which shows marked notching or slurring (Figs. 10–1 and 10–2).

Interestingly, there is little delay in the initial portion of the QRS complex because hyperkalemia has less slowing effect on conduction in the Purkinje fibers than in muscle cells. Because of the delay in ventricular activation the frontal plane axis usually shifts to the left. The slow activation of the ventricles leads to repolarization of earlier activated areas while other myocardial cells are still being depolarized. This results in merging of the wide QRS and the tall peaked T waves. The decrease in conduction velocity in the atrium leads to wide, low-voltage P waves with a prolonged PR interval (Fig. 10–2). A further increase in potassium leads to disappearance of the P waves (Fig. 10–3).

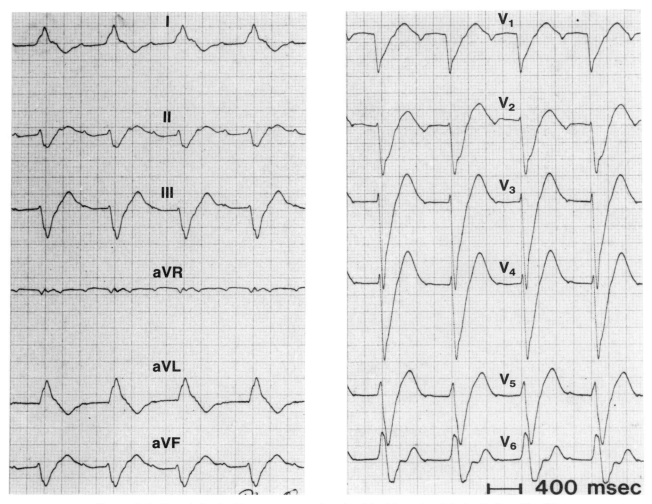

Figure 10–2. Hyperkalemia. The serum potassium level in this patient is 7.6 mEq/liter. The PR is prolonged, as is the QRS duration; there is left axis deviation, and the S wave moves steeply into the T wave without an isoelectric ST segment.

TREATMENT

Mild Hyperkalemia

Determine the cause (usually renal disease). Correct, if possible, the underlying disease.

Severe Hyperkalemia

1. Give an IV infusion of 10 to 30 ml of calcium gluconate (10 percent) over 1 to 5 minutes with constant ECG monitoring. Calcium infusions do not lower plasma potassium concentrations; they do, however, immediately but transiently alter the effect of potassium on the cell membrane.

2. Give 200 to 500 ml of hypertonic glucose solution (10 percent) in 30 minutes, and 500 to 1000 ml over the next several hours. Glucose decreases the effect of potassium toxicity by shifting potassium into the cells.

3. Sodium bicarbonate (2 to 3 ampuls) may be added to 1 L of 5 percent dextrose in 0.9 percent saline. Sodium bicarbonate helps to shift potassium into the cells even in patients who are not acidotic.

4. Give cation exchange resins (sodium polystyrene sulfonate) by retention enema; this may be repeated until potassium levels are within safe limits. Give oral doses of 20 gm 3 or 4 times a day together with 20 ml of 70 percent sorbitol solution.

5. In case of renal failure, initiate hemodialysis or peritoneal dialysis along with one of the treatments above.

Figure 10–3 illustrates the 12-lead ECG before and after treatment for severe hyperkalemia. The serum potassium was 8.6 mEq/L in the 12-lead ECG on the left. The ECG on the right shows the disappearance of the hyperkalemic ECG abnormalities as the potassium level is restored to normal.

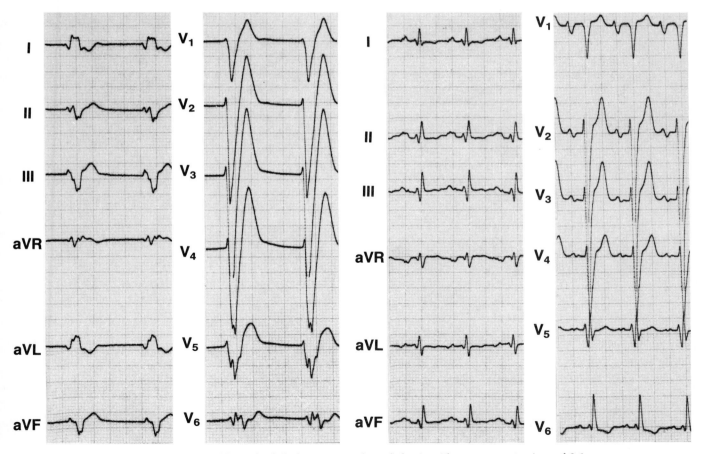

Figure 10–3. The ECG on the left shows severe hyperkalemia with a serum potassium of 8.6 mEq/liter. The ECG on the right was taken following treatment. Note that the P wave has returned, the QRS duration is less, and that the QRS complex and the T wave are separated.

HYPOKALEMIA

MECHANISM

Hypokalemia promotes the occurrence of early afterdepolarizations (see also Chapter 9), which may lead to the emergence of torsade de pointes arrhythmias. It also causes arrhythmias due to enhanced automaticity.

In progressive hypokalemia the cell membrane becomes less and less negative until the cell is eventually nonexcitable. Moreover, if digitalis is administered when the extracellular potassium is low, arrhythmogenicity is likely to be promoted.[4]

Digitalis and potassium compete for membrane binding sites, and with lowered potassium in the extracellular fluid, more digitalis binds to the potassium position on the membrane sodium-potassium ATPase, augmenting digitalis toxicity.

ECG CHANGES IN PROGRESSIVE HYPOKALEMIA

1. Progressive ST depression
2. Decrease in T wave amplitude

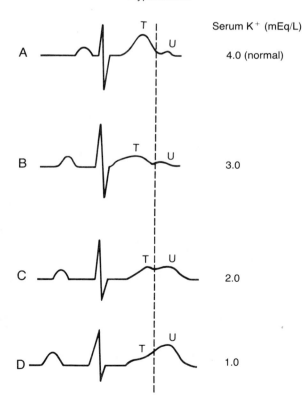

Figure 10–4. A representation of the progressive T and U wave changes in hypokalemia. The normal ECG has a small U wave of the same polarity as the T wave (serum potassium 3.5 to 4.5 mEq/L). When the serum potassium level decreases there is a lowering in amplitude of the T wave, whereas amplitude of the U wave increases. At very low serum potassium levels the U wave fuses with the T wave and becomes dominant. (From Conover, M.: Understanding Electrocardiography. St. Louis, 1988, CV Mosby.)

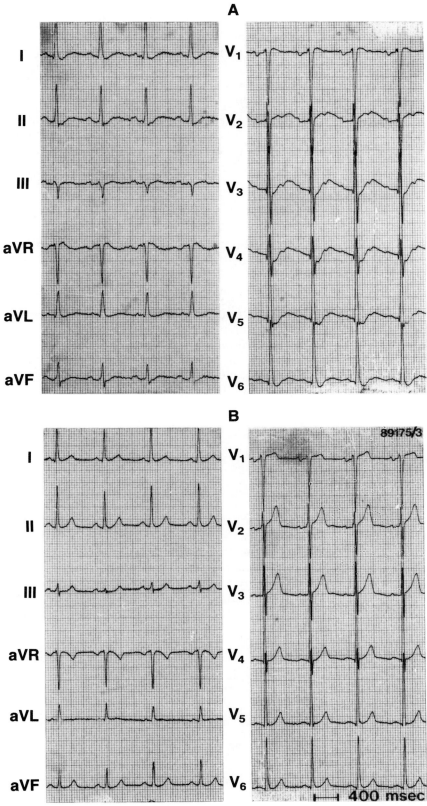

Figure 10–5. (*A*) A 12-lead ECG from a patient with hypokalemia (serum potassium of 1.47 mEq/ L). Note the giant U wave, which is best seen in the precordial leads V_2 to V_6. (*B*) The ECG of the same patient after correction of hypokalemia.

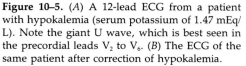

3. Increase in U wave amplitude; in advanced stages the T and U are fused.
4. In advanced hypokalemia the QRS amplitude and duration increase.
5. P wave amplitude and duration are usually increased.
6. PR interval is usually slightly prolonged.

Figure 10–4 is a schematic representation of the typical T and U wave changes associated with progressive hypokalemia; the tracing in Figure 10–5 is from a patient with a serum potassium of 1.47 mEq/L. Note that the U wave has fused with the T wave (best seen in leads V_2 to V_6) and is larger than the T wave.

TREATMENT

Determine the underlying cause. Usually fluid and potassium loss induced by severe diarrhea or potassium-losing diuretics is responsible. Occasionally, other causes can be found, such as use of a liquid protein diet (to lose weight) or frequent ingestion of licorice.

1. In severe potassium deficiency give intravenous potassium chloride (40 to 60 mEq/L at 20 mEq/hour; approximately 200 to 250 mEq/day).
2. Perform continuous ECG monitoring.
3. If torsade de pointes ventricular arrhythmias are present, see Chapter 9 for rapid control of the arrhythmia.
4. In moderate hypokalemia give potassium salts by mouth.

Figure 10–5 shows the 12-lead ECG of a patient during severe hypokalemia and following treatment.

SUMMARY

Severe hyperkalemia is marked by a broad QRS, bradycardia, left axis deviation, loss of P wave and ST segment, and tall tented T waves. The emergency treatment of hyperkalemia includes calcium gluconate, hypertonic glucose solution, sodium bicarbonate, and cation exchange resins.

Severe hypokalemia is marked by ST segment depression, decrease in T wave amplitude, and increase in U wave amplitude. The emergency treatment of hypokalemia is intravenous and oral potassium chloride.

References

1. Hylander, B.: Survival of extreme hyperkalemia. Acta Med. Scand. 221:121–123, 1987.
2. Winkler, A.W., Hoff, H.E., and Smith, P.K.: Electrocardiographic changes and concentration of potassium in serum following intravenous injection of potassium chloride. Am. J. Physiol. 124:478–485, 1938.
3. Bryant, G.M.: Effect of potassium on ventricular deflections of the electrocardiogram in hypertensive cardiovascular disease. Proc. Soc. Exp. Biol. Med. 7:557–558, 1948.
4. Suki, W.N., and Jackson, D.: Hypokalemia—cause and treatment. Heart Lung 7:854–860, 1978.

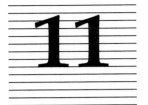

Pacing Emergencies

EMERGENCY APPROACH

EARLY FAILURE TO CAPTURE AND SENSE

1. If failure to capture, increase the output (amplitude or pulse width).
2. If unsuccessful, reposition the electrode catheter.
3. If failure to sense, increase the sensitivity; when sensing is still inadequate, change to unipolar sensing.
4. If unsuccessful, reposition the catheter.

PACING FAILURE

1. If no pacemaker spikes are present, inspect all conducting wires and connections; record an ECG from each electrode.
2. If there are intermittent pacemaker spikes, only one electrode may be involved; convert to a unipolar system.

PACEMAKER SYNDROME

1. Prevent the pacemaker syndrome by carefully checking for the presence of ventriculoatrial (VA) conduction during temporary pacemaker insertion; be aware that large hearts and hearts with thick ventricular muscles (as in hypertension) require atrial contribution for adequate systolic output.
2. If pacemaker syndrome is first recognized after implantation, program the rate so that the majority of beats are spontaneous.
3. If unsuccessful, reoperation is necessary for conversion to an atrial pacing device in case of intact atrioventricular (AV) conduction or to a dual chamber unit in case of AV block.

MYOCARDIAL PERFORATION

1. To confirm myocardial perforation, record a unipolar electrogram from the pacing electrode(s); an ECG showing QRS and T waves similar to those recorded on precordial lead V_3 or V_4 indicates that the electrode is outside the heart.
2. Gently withdraw the pacing catheter while recording the ECG from the electrode; in case of a bipolar catheter use the distal electrode! When the QRS complex and T wave are opposite to lead V_3 or V_4, the distal electrode is again inside the right ventricle.

3. In the event of pericardial tamponade, immediate pericardiocentesis and drainage are indicated.
4. Closely monitor the patient.
5. Discontinue anticoagulants.

PACEMAKER-MEDIATED TACHYCARDIA

1. Reprogram the atrial sensing refractory period so that retrograde atrial signals are not sensed.
2. Decrease atrial sensing sensitivity.
3. Program a short AV interval.
4. Or switch to a DVI mode; this eliminates atrial sensing and terminates the tachycardia.

THROMBOSIS AND PULMONARY EMBOLISM

Heparin and thrombolytic therapy is usually sufficient for clinically important thrombosis.

INFECTION OR EROSION OF THE PULSE GENERATOR

1. A temporary pacemaker is inserted, the entire permanent pacing unit is removed, and a new unit is installed on the contralateral side.
2. The removal of the involved lead is usually difficult, and continuous careful traction is applied to the lead.
3. If this fails, in cases of endocarditis, thoracotomy may be necessary.
4. The lead may be saved in the case of pacemaker erosion if the condition is detected early.

ELECTROMYOGRAPHIC INHIBITION (EMI)

1. Decrease the sensitivity of the pacemaker.
2. If unsuccessful, reprogram the pacemaker from a unipolar to a bipolar unit.
3. If unsuccessful, reoperation may be necessary.

EMERGENCY TEMPORARY PACING

Prepare for emergency temporary pacing in the event of:

1. Complete AV block with a slow ventricular escape rhythm
2. Symptomatic sinus bradycardia, asystole, or prolonged sinus pauses
3. Acute anterior myocardial infarction with complete heart block, right bundle branch block (RBBB) or left bundle branch block (LBBB) with type II second-degree AV block or RBBB with new hemiblock
4. Acute inferior myocardial infarction with complete heart block leading to hypotension, congestive heart failure, or ventricular arrhythmias
5. Bradycardia-induced or drug-induced torsade de pointes
6. Malfunction of a permanent pacemaker
7. Digitalis toxicity-induced ventricular tachycardia (VT) being treated with drugs (e.g., Dilantin) that suppress impulse formation
8. Consider use of temporary pacing in case of tachycardias that do not respond to antiarrhythmic drug therapy; these include sustained VT, AV nodal tachycardia, and atrial flutter. In these patients the arrhythmia frequently can be terminated by pacing-induced premature stimuli or pacing above the tachycardia rate.

EARLY FAILURE TO CAPTURE AND SENSE

In a small percentage of patients, early failure to capture or sense may occur during the first days following pacemaker implantation and may be corrected by adjusting the output amplitude, pulse width, or sensitivity. If this is unsuccessful, reoperation with repositioning may be indicated.

MECHANISM

Catheter Dislodgement

The most common cause of failure to capture or sense is dislodgement of the catheter. Catheter dislodgement may or may not be seen on radiographs, depending upon the degree of catheter displacement. When the magnitude of the pacemaker deflection is adequate, failure to capture usually indicates catheter dislodgement. In case of a spontaneous rhythm faster than the selected pacing rate, the intracardiac electrode transmits a signal of 2 mV or more to the generator's sensing circuit. This signal inhibits the output of the pacemaker and resets the pacing cycle. If the catheter displacement results in an intracardiac signal of less than 2 mV, premature ventricular complexes (PVCs) and/or the patient's own rhythm will no longer be sensed and the pacemaker no longer acts in the demand mode but performs like a fixed-rate pacemaker, discharging regardless of PVCs or the patient's own rhythm. This is a dangerous situation in patients whose fibrillatory threshold is lowered because of acute myocardial ischemia, digitalis toxicity, or electrolyte imbalance.

Types of Malsensing

Continuous Subsensing. None of the spontaneous QRS complexes is sensed, leading to fixed-rate pacing.

Intermittent Malsensing. If the catheter moves in the cardiac cavity, some spontaneous cardiac signals may generate sufficient voltage to be sensed and others not. This leads to intermittent sensing problems.

Oversensing. Occasionally the T wave may generate sufficient voltage to be misinterpreted by the sensing system as a QRS complex. Oversensing will result in suppression of pacemaker activity.

Sensing Misinterpretation

In some cases, sensing failure is really sensing misinterpretation. For example, the development of RBBB causes a delay in propagation of the impulse to the right ventricle where the electrode is located. This is perceived by the electrode sensing unit as inactivity, and the pacemaker spike appears in the spontaneous QRS complex (fusion or pseudofusion).

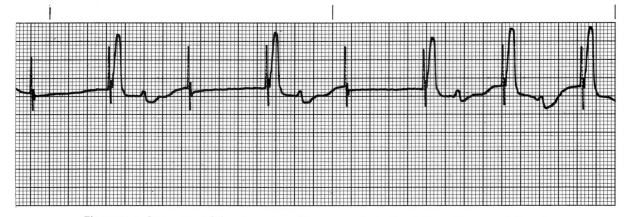

Figure 11–1. Intermittent failure to capture. Note pacemaker spikes 1, 3, and 5 are not followed by ventricular complexes although the ventricles are nonrefractory.

ECG RECOGNITION

Figure 11–1 is an example of intermittent failure to capture.

Figure 11–2 illustrates failure to sense. In this tracing, the pacemaker fails to sense the patient's own rhythm and fires on the T waves of four complexes until finally it captures the heart.

TREATMENT

Since the threshold for capture can change with time, changes in body position, and minor shifts in electrode location, capture may be restored by simply increasing the output (amplitude or pulse width); failure to sense may be corrected by increasing the sensitivity.

If the sensing failure is due to a dislodgement of the catheter, increasing the sensitivity may solve the problem. If this does not help, the permanent pacemaker should be converted from the demand mode to fixed-rate mode until the problem is corrected with reoperation and repositioning.

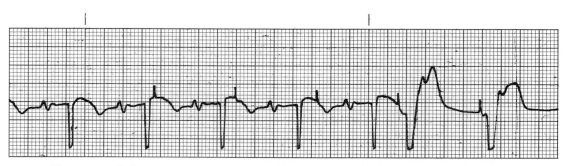

Figure 11–2. Failure to sense. The pacemaker fails to sense the patient's intrinsic rhythm and fires on T waves.

In summary:

1. If failure to capture, increase the output (mA or pulse width).
2. If unsuccessful, early reoperation is indicated, with repositioning of the permanent pacemaker.
3. If failure to sense, increase the sensitivity.
4. If unsuccessful in case of a permanent pacemaker, convert the demand mode to fixed-rate mode and prepare for reoperation.
5. If unsuccessful in case of a temporary pacemaker, reposition the catheter.

PACING FAILURE

Failure to pace may result in profound bradycardia and requires immediate intervention. Reoperation correcting the appropriate component is usually indicated.

MECHANISM

Late failure to pace may be related to change in myocardial threshold, battery depletion, or failure of the lead or pacemaker components. These conditions may or may not require reoperation. Noninvasive diagnosis of the problem using the information obtained with telemetry is now possible with the newer pacemakers.

ECG RECOGNITION AND TREATMENT

If there are no pacemaker spikes, a break in the system anywhere from the lead to the pulse generator is suspected. In case of a temporary pacemaker, all conducting wires and connections should be inspected and electrograms recorded from each electrode.

Intermittent activity indicates wire fracture. It may be that only one of the electrodes of a bipolar system is involved. If so, conversion to unipolar pacing should be done until the catheter can be replaced.

PACEMAKER SYNDROME

The pacemaker syndrome is a complex of symptoms related to adverse hemodynamic effects of single-chamber ventricular pacing.

MECHANISM

This syndrome is most common in patients with sick sinus syndrome who have intact VA conduction during ventricular pacing. Symptoms are the result of variations in cardiac output and blood pressure due to nonsynchronization of atrial and ventricular contraction. Contraction of the atrium against a closed mitral valve leads to a decrease in left ventricular filling, which in turn causes a lesser stroke volume and a lower blood pressure.[1]

ECG RECOGNITION AND PHYSICAL FINDINGS

The ECG typically shows independent beating of the atria and ventricles or VA conduction following the paced complexes.

The symptoms include fatigue, dizziness, syncope, and pulmonary congestion. The diagnosis is made by the history alone or by observation of fluctuation in peripheral blood pressure and cannon A waves in the neck.

TREATMENT

1. During pacemaker insertion, prevent the syndrome by carefully checking for VA conduction. Be aware that large hearts and hearts with thickened ventricular muscle are especially in need of an appropriately timed atrial contraction for optimal cardiac output.
2. If pacemaker syndrome is first recognized after pacemaker implantation, lower the ventricular paced rate so that the majority of beats are conducted sinus beats.
3. If unsuccessful, reoperation may be indicated for conversion to an atrial pacing device in case of intact AV conduction or a dual chamber unit in case of AV block.

PACEMAKER-MEDIATED (OR PACEMAKER CIRCUS MOVEMENT) TACHYCARDIA

Pacemaker-mediated tachycardia may occur in patients with intact VA conduction after implantation of an atrial synchronized, ventricular inhibited (VDD), or AV universal (DDD) pacemaker.[2]

MECHANISM

The tachycardia begins following retrograde conduction of a P wave from a ventricular beat, either paced or spontaneous. The retrograde P wave is then sensed by the atrial electrode. The ventricular pacemaker waits for the programmed AV interval and then fires. Again, retrograde conduction occurs to the atria followed by paced ventricular activation. This repetitive tachycardia is comparable to that seen in patients having an accessory AV pathway. As long as the retrogradely conducted impulses reach the atrium after the pacemaker atrial refractory period has ended, tachycardia persists at a rate equal to or near the programmed atrial rate limit. Whether or not the retrograde P wave is sensed by the atrial circuit depends upon the length of the refractory period of the atrial sensing amplifier.

ECG RECOGNITION

1. The tachycardia is paroxysmal.
2. The P wave during the tachycardia is retrograde (negative in leads II, III, and aVF).
3. The PR interval during tachycardia is the same as the PR interval during sinus rhythm due to the fact that there is a programmed AV interval.
4. The QRS complex of the tachycardia is a paced complex.

Figure 11–3 is an ECG tracing of a pacemaker circus movement tachycardia. A retrograde P wave follows the PVC. The atrial electrode senses

DDD AV Interval 150ms   Upper Rate 150bpm

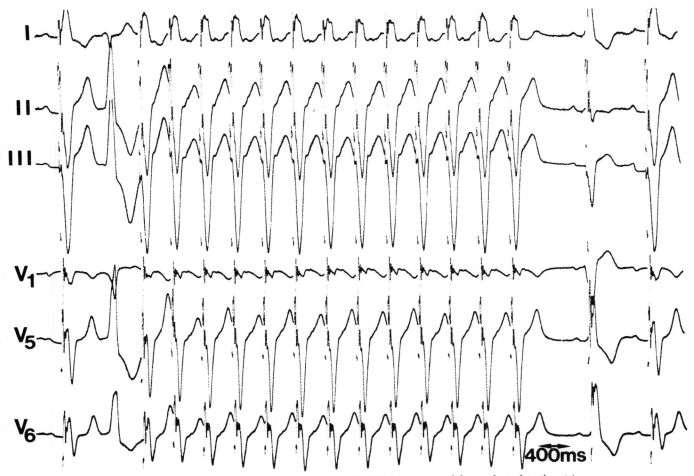

Figure 11–3. Pacemaker-mediated tachycardia. The VPC is retrogradely conducted to the atria. The atrial electrode senses the retrograde P wave. This is followed by ventricular stimulation after the programmed AV delay. Every paced ventricular complex is followed by retrograde conduction to the atria. The tachycardia terminates spontaneously because of retrograde VA block.

this impulse and activates the ventricular pacemaker. Every subsequently paced ventricular beat is then retrogradely conducted to the atrium, leading to atrial sensing followed by ventricular pacing. This repetitive sequence sustains the tachycardia until VA block occurs.

TREATMENT

1. Prolong the atrial sensing refractory period so that retrograde atrial signals fall within that refractory period.
2. Decrease atrial sensing sensitivity.
3. Program a short AV interval, thereby preventing VA conduction of the ventricular paced beat.
4. Or, switch to a DVI mode; this eliminates atrial sensing and terminates the tachycardia.

MYOCARDIAL PERFORATION AND TAMPONADE

Myocardial perforation by the pacing electrode may require gentle withdrawal of the pacing catheter. Pericardial tamponade is extremely rare and requires immediate pericardiocentesis and drainage.

ECG RECOGNITION AND PHYSICAL FINDINGS

Myocardial perforation is suggested by loss of capture, intercostal or diaphragmatic stimulation, and the occurrence of a pericardial friction rub.

Confirm perforation by recording a unipolar electrogram from the pacing electrode. In case of a bipolar electrode, record from the distal electrode. An electrogram with a positive R wave, mimicking a lead V_3 or V_4, suggests perforation. A unipolar electrogram is recorded by connecting one of the V leads to the electrode of the catheter. If the electrode is situated in the right ventricular apex, the QRS complex is negative and the ST segment elevated (Fig. 11–4B). If the myocardium has been perforated and the electrode is situated within the pericardial sac, the QRS is more positive and the T wave is opposite to the intracavitary T wave (Fig. 11–4A). In case of perforation, the ECG from the electrode is similar to the precordial lead V_3 or V_4.

An echocardiogram may confirm the diagnosis.

TREATMENT

1. If myocardial perforation is the diagnosis, gently withdraw the pacing catheter.
2. In the event of pericardial tamponade, immediate pericardiocentesis and drainage are indicated.
3. Closely monitor the patient.
4. Discontinue any anticoagulants.

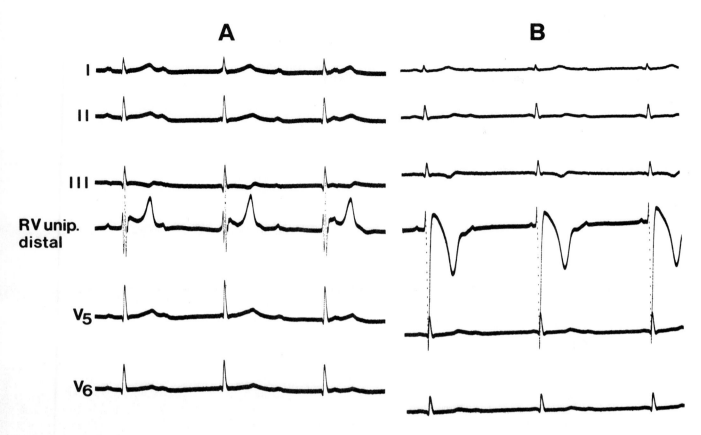

A

B

I

II

III

**RV unip.
distal**

V₅

V₆

after catheter repositioning

Figure 11–4. ECG from the electrode catheter in myocardial perforation. The distal unipolar recording from the RV electrode catheter in *panel A* shows an R/S ratio of the QRS of about 1 and T wave polarity similar to the precordial leads V_5 and V_6. After withdrawal of the catheter the electrogram shows the typical right ventricular endocavitary complex (R/S ratio less than 1, negative T wave).

THROMBOSIS AND PULMONARY EMBOLISM

Evidence of mild venous thrombosis has been reported in up to 30 percent of patients with pacemakers. Serious thrombosis of the subclavian and axillary veins may occur in up to 2 percent of patients.

Pulmonary embolism secondary to right atrial or right ventricular thrombus on a pacing wire may occur. The ECG recognition of acute pulmonary embolism can be found in Chapter 7.

TREATMENT

Therapy with heparin and a thrombolytic agent is usually sufficient for clinically significant thrombosis.

INFECTION OR EROSION OF THE PULSE GENERATOR

Permanent pacemaker implantation may be complicated by early and late infections. *Staphylococcus aureus* is the most common organism in early infections, and *Staphylococcus epidermidis* the most common in late infections. On rare occasions permanent pacemakers may erode through the skin. Reoperation is required to remove the pacemaker and insert a new one in a different location.[3, 4]

TREATMENT

When infection of the pulse generator pocket occurs, it is almost always necessary to remove the entire unit. In general, medical therapy alone is unsatisfactory and surgical removal of the entire pacing system, interim use of a temporary pacemaker, and placement of a new unit on the contralateral side are recommended. In some cases without bacteremia, explantation and implantation of the new unit may be accomplished in the course of one operation. Removal of a chronically implanted lead is generally difficult and has been made more difficult by use of active fixation leads. The basic technique involves continuous careful traction applied to the lead once it is dissected from all its attachments. Continuous traction by means of 1-pound weights has been employed. If all these means fail, thoracotomy may be necessary.

With pacemaker erosion, if detected early, the lead may be saved. It may be possible to isolate the lead in a relatively proximal position and attach a new coupling device. The pacemaker generator is removed, the eroded pocket is closed, and the new pacemaker pack is placed in another location on the same side.

ELECTROMYOGRAPHIC INHIBITION

MECHANISM

The electrical potentials generated by pectoral muscles around the pulse generator of a unipolar inhibitory pacemaker may inhibit the pulse generator in as many as one-third of all unipolar pacemakers implanted. This inhibition causes symptoms in approximately one-half of those affected. Myopotentials may also cause false triggering in DDD units due to pacemaker interpretation of myopotentials as P waves. In new pacemakers, the electrical potentials from muscle activity are rejected due to improved filtering in the circuitry.[5]

ECG RECOGNITION

Figure 11–5 is a tracing from a Holter monitor lead, demonstrating myopotential inhibition of a demand pacemaker. Note that the pectoral muscle

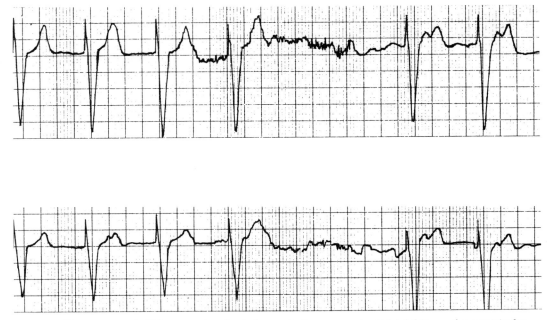

Figure 11–5. A Holter monitor lead demonstrating myopotential inhibition of a ventricular demand pacemaker. (From Jacobs, L.J., Kerzner, J.S., Diamond, M.A., et al.: Pacemaker inhibition by myopotentials determined by Holter monitoring. PACE 5:30–33, 1982.)

potentials are picked up by the surface ECG and appear as an artifact. There are no pacemaker spikes during this time.

You may test for the possibility of electromyopotential inhibition by having the patient raise a weight or press the hands together forcefully during ECG monitoring.

TREATMENT

Most pacemakers have an interference rate to which they revert if exposed to input signals above a rate determined by the manufacturer (usually 300/ minute). The interference rate is an asynchronous fixed-rate mode, which may be the same as the automatic rate but is usually faster. If this is not the case, the following steps may relieve the problem:

1. Decrease the sensitivity of the pacemaker.
2. Most pacemakers can be reprogrammed from a unipolar to a bipolar unit.
3. If unsuccessful, reoperation may be necessary.

ARRHYTHMIAS DURING PACEMAKER INSERTION

During insertion of the pacing lead, atrial or ventricular arrhythmias may occur as a result of catheter manipulation. If ventricular fibrillation results, defibrillate immediately.

References

1. Ausubel, K., and Furman, S.: The pacemaker syndrome. Ann. Intern. Med. 103:420–429, 1985.
2. Den Dulk, K., Lindeman, F.W., Bär, F.W., et al.: Pacemaker related tachycardia. PACE 5:476–485, 1982.
3. Choo, M.H., Holmes, D.R., Gersh, B., et al.: Permanent pacemaker infections: Characterization and management. Am. J. Cardiol. 48:559–564, 1981.
4. Lewis, A.B., Hayes, D.L., Holmes, D.K., et al.: Update on infections involving permanent pacemakers: Characterization and management. J. Thorac. Cardiovasc. Surg. 89:758–763, 1985.
5. Barold, S.S., Falkoff, M.D., Ong, L.S., et al.: Diaphragmatic myopotential inhibition in multiprogrammable unipolar and bipolar pulse generators. In Steinbach (ed.): Cardiac Pacing. Darmstadt, 1983, Steinkoff Verlag, pp. 537–540.

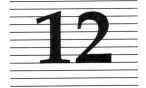

C H A P T E R

12

Prehospital Cardiac Emergencies

It is now possible for paramedics to obtain a 12-lead ECG in the field and to transmit that record to the hospital by cellular phone. This allows early physician consultation and rapid institution of treatment.

Early thrombolytic therapy started outside the hospital may reduce the size of myocardial infarction, thereby improving survival.[1, 2] Also, the correct identification and early treatment of patients with pulmonary embolism or a tachycardia can be lifesaving. To obtain optimal results, the paramedic should be well trained in history-taking and familiar with the ECG recognition of cardiac emergencies.

CHEST PAIN WITH ST SEGMENT ELEVATION ON THE ECG

There is no longer discussion about the value of early thrombolytic therapy after an acute myocardial infarction (MI). The earlier the treatment is started the better, especially in patients with large infarctions. It is likely therefore that paramedics have an increasingly important role in the early administration of thrombolytic therapy, making it mandatory that they be able to recognize those patients likely to benefit from that therapy.

PROCEDURE FOR INITIAL EVALUATION

1. Transmit a 12-lead ECG to the base hospital; evaluate ECG criteria governing the decision to initiate thrombolytic treatment. (See Chapter 1.)

   If inferior wall MI is revealed, record a V_4R lead to identify those patients having an occlusion high in the right coronary artery.

   If anterior wall MI is apparent, evaluate 12 leads for the extent of infarction by counting the number of precordial leads showing ST segment elevation and the amount of ST elevation.

   Know how to recognize bundle branch block.

2. Take a history of chest pain. Report these findings to the hospital to

further identify candidates for thrombolytic therapy and to rule out those for whom thrombolysis is contraindicated.

3. Measure blood pressure.
4. Review again inclusion and exclusion criteria.
5. Report findings to the physician at the base hospital, including your own ECG evaluation; thereafter, the decision is made to withhold or proceed with thrombolytic therapy.
6. If thrombolytics are indicated:

   • An informed consent may be necessary; this should be read to the patient.
   • Initiate thrombolysis.
   • Begin transport.
   • Record time pain began; decision time, type and amount of thrombolytic agent given; and hospital arrival time.

HISTORY-TAKING FOR CHEST PAIN

1. How long have you had your pain? (More than 15 minutes, less than 2 hours, less than 4 hours?)
2. Please point to where your pain is located. (Sternal; precordial, left chest; right chest; epigastrium/lower or midchest? Specify if another location.)
3. How would you describe your pain? (If possible, this should be in the patient's own words without suggestions from the examiner.) The pain may be sharp, dull, aching, like a weight on or in the chest, burning, tightness, or ripping.
4. What makes your pain less? What makes it worse? (Sitting up, leaning forward, lying flat, belching, vomiting, walking, nothing?)
5. Does your pain radiate to another area? (Shoulder; jaw; neck, arm or arms?)
6. Have you been sweating?
7. Are you short of breath?
8. Did you use nitroglycerin? (Sublingual or patch?)
9. Have you been nauseated or vomiting?
10. In the past, have you had a heart attack, angina, coronary bypass, peripheral artery bypass?
11. Do you smoke or have high blood pressure, diabetes mellitus, high blood cholesterol, or a family history of heart attacks or sudden death?

PHYSICAL EXAMINATION

The physical examination is performed in order to be informed about the pump function of the heart and the blood supply to the extremities.

1. Describe general appearance. (Pale, cyanotic, sweating, hemiparetic, lethargic, status of peripheral perfusion?)
2. Record the blood pressure and pulse rate.
3. Is there jugular venous distention?
4. Can bruits be heard over the carotids?

5. Lungs clear? Rales?
6. Heart (Regular, irregular, murmurs, S3 gallop, pericardial friction rub?)
7. Abdomen (Tender, tense, pulsatile mass?)
8. Evaluate mental status for recent change.
9. Weakness of arms and/or legs of recent onset?

CONTRAINDICATIONS TO THROMBOLYTIC THERAPY

A history of cerebral disease like stroke, seizures, brain surgery, brain tumor
Thoracic or abdominal aneurysm
Pregnancy
Bleeding (menstrual, gastrointestinal, or genitourinary)
Surgery in the past 2 months
Terminal cancer
Kidney disease
Liver disease
Diabetes
Colitis
Crohn's enteritis

CANDIDATES FOR THROMBOLYSIS

In order to qualify for thrombolytic therapy the patient should have a qualifying 12-lead ECG (described below) and should:

1. Be oriented and cooperative
2. Have had pain for more than 15 minutes
3. Have a systolic blood pressure of more than 80 and less than 200 mmHg
4. Have a systolic blood pressure difference between right and left arms of less than 30 mmHg and diastolic of less than 20 mmHg

ECG CRITERIA FOR DECISION TO INITIATE THROMBOLYSIS

Information Needed

1. Time from onset of pain (less than 2 hours, 2–4 hours, more than 4 hours)
2. Presence or absence of Q waves
3. Type of MI (anterior or inferior)
4. ST score

How to Calculate ST Score

High ST Score. This is a sum of more than 12 mm elevation in the precordial leads in anterior MI or more than 7 mm in leads II, III, and aVF in inferior MI.

Low ST Score. This is a sum of less than 12 mm elevation in the precordial leads in anterior MI or less than 7 mm in leads II, III, and aVF in inferior MI. (See also Chapter 1.)

Keep in mind: The shorter the time interval from onset of chest pain to recording of the ECG, and the higher the ST score, the more heart muscle can be saved by thrombolysis (see Chapter 1).

EVALUATION OF LEAD V₄R IN ACUTE INFERIOR MYOCARDIAL INFARCTION

Lead V_4R is useful to:

- Identify patients having a large inferior MI
- Determine whether right ventricular MI has occurred
- Identify a patient who is at high risk for developing AV block
- Identify the location of the coronary artery occlusion in the event intracoronary thrombolysis is indicated (see Chapter 1)

ECG RECOGNITION OF BUNDLE BRANCH BLOCK IN ACUTE ANTERIOR WALL MYOCARDIAL INFARCTION

In acute anterior wall MI, bundle branch block (BBB) is an ominous finding. In such a case the physician should be prepared for aggressive therapy when the patient arrives in the hospital. It is therefore important for this information to be transmitted to the base hospital. The paramedic should also be able to recognize these conditions. The ECG signs of BBB with and without MI are discussed in Chapter 1.

CHEST PAIN WITH ST SEGMENT DEPRESSION OR T WAVE INVERSION

1. Take a history and do a physical examination.
2. Obtain a 12-lead ECG and transmit to the base hospital.
3. Evaluate the ECG for signs of critical proximal left anterior descending coronary artery (LAD) stenosis and for left mainstem and three-vessel disease (see also Chapter 2), both of which are indications for rapid cardiac catheterization and revascularization therapy. Especially at risk are patients showing these ECG findings in the presence of a low blood pressure!
4. Transmit your findings to the base hospital.

ECG RECOGNITION OF LEFT MAINSTEM AND THREE-VESSEL DISEASE

- Unstable angina (see also Chapter 2)
- ST elevation in leads aVR and V_1
- ST depression in eight or more leads

ECG RECOGNITION OF CRITICAL PROXIMAL LEFT ANTERIOR DESCENDING CORONARY ARTERY STENOSIS

Unstable angina

No pathological precordial Q waves

ST segment isoelectric or minimally elevated (1 mm), concave or straight symmetrical T wave inversion (This may begin with very slight negativity at the terminal part of the T wave in leads V_1 to V_3.)

Whereas the ECG changes of left mainstem and three-vessel disease are typically present *during* pain, those of critical proximal LAD stenosis usually develop *after* chest pain has subsided.

CONSCIOUS PATIENT IN TACHYCARDIA

1. Record a 12-lead ECG and transmit to the base hospital.
2. Obtain vital signs and evaluate neck veins for cannon A waves (AV dissociation) or for the "frog sign" (supraventricular tachycardia [SVT]).
3. Divide patients according to those having a narrow (<0.12 sec) or a broad (≥0.12 sec) QRS tachycardia.
4. If broad QRS tachycardia is present, remain calm, determine if lead V_1 is positive or negative, and apply morphological rules to differentiate SVT from ventricular tachycardia (VT) (see Chapter 3). Systematically evaluate the 12-lead ECG, and examine your patient for physical signs of AV dissociation (a sign of VT). If in doubt, *do not give verapamil;* give procainamide.

PHYSICAL SIGNS OF SUPRAVENTRICULAR TACHYCARDIA

Pulse. Regular in regular SVT.

Blood Pressure. Constant in regular SVT.

First Heart Sound. Constant in regular SVT. Pulse, blood pressure, and loudness of the first heart sound will vary in atrial fibrillation and atrial flutter with changing AV conduction.

Neck Veins. In atrial flutter, flutter waves; in AV nodal reentry and circus movement tachycardia (CMT), the "frog sign" (see p. 76).

EFFECT OF CAROTID SINUS MASSAGE ON SUPRAVENTRICULAR TACHYCARDIA

Know how to perform this maneuver (see Chapter 4). The gag reflex is an excellent vagal maneuver and substitute for carotid sinus massage, which is usually performed by the physician.

Sinus Tachycardia. Gradual and temporary, slowing heart rate.

Atrial Tachycardia. Cessation or temporary slowing (AV block) of tachycardia or no effect.

Atrial Flutter. Temporary slowing (AV block), conversion to atrial fibrillation, or no effect.

Atrial Fibrillation. Temporary slowing (AV block) or no effect.

AV Nodal Reentry Tachycardia. Cessation of tachycardia or no effect.

Circus Movement Tachycardia Using an Accessory AV Pathway. Cessation of tachycardia or no effect.

PHYSICAL SIGNS OF VENTRICULAR TACHYCARDIA (IN CASE OF AV DISSOCIATION)

Blood Pressure. Beat-to-beat changes in systolic blood pressure.

First Heart Sound. Varying loudness of the first heart sound.

Neck Veins. Irregular cannon A waves in the jugular venous pulse.

EVALUATION OF THE ECG

In Lead V_1-Positive Broad QRS Tachycardia

SVT is most likely in case of a triphasic pattern in lead V_1 (rSR'); VT is most likely with a monophasic or biphasic pattern in lead V_1. The "rabbit ear" clue is also an indication of VT (two peaks in lead V_1 with the left peak taller). When lead V_1 is not diagnostic, look at lead V_6. A triphasic pattern (qRS) in lead V_6 suggests SVT, whereas a deep S (R/S ratio of <1) or QS indicates VT (see Chapter 3).

In Lead V_1-Negative Broad QRS Tachycardia

The following findings in leads V_1, V_2, and V_6 are highly predictive of VT:

1. A broad R of 0.04 sec or more in lead V_1 or V_2
2. A notched or slurred downstroke on the S or QS wave in lead V_1 or V_2
3. A distance of 0.07 sec or more from the onset of the ventricular complex to the nadir of the QS or S in lead V_1 or V_2
4. Any Q in lead V_6 strongly suggests VT, but *only* if the complex is mainly negative in lead V_1; this clue cannot be applied to the tachycardia that is positive in lead V_1.

In SVT with left bundle branch block (LBBB) aberration, if there is an r wave it is narrow and sharp in lead V_1 and/or lead V_2 and the S wave has a clean, swift downstroke (see Chapter 3). If the recording from lead V_1 looks like VT, it is treated as VT; but if the recording from lead V_1 looks like SVT, be sure to check leads V_2 and V_6 before deciding.

OTHER HELPFUL ECG CLUES THAT INDICATE VENTRICULAR TACHYCARDIA

1. AV dissociation
2. QRS width more than 0.14 sec favors VT (except in the case of digitalis toxicity or in the presence of drugs that slow intraventricular conduction).
3. Fusion beats, capture beats, and precordial concordance (all precordial leads showing either a completely positive or negative QRS complex) also favor a diagnosis of VT.

TREATMENT

If Ventricular Tachycardia

Administer IV procainamide 10 mg/kg body weight IV over 5 minutes; or lidocaine 1 mg/kg body weight IV if an acute MI is suspected. (In nonischemic VT, procainamide is more effective than lidocaine.)
　　　If unsuccessful, cardiovert.
　　　Obtain a history regarding frequency of tachycardia episodes and complaints during an attack of tachycardia.

If Supraventricular Tachycardia With Aberration

Transmit the 12-lead ECG to the base hospital; the following may be ordered:
　　　Vagal stimulation
　　　Adenosine 6-mg bolus (12 mg may be repeated twice) or verapamil 10 mg IV over 3 minutes; if unsuccessful:
　　　Procainamide 10 mg/kg body weight IV over 5 minutes
　　　If unsuccessful, cardiovert.

If In Doubt

Do *not* give verapamil; on advice of physician give IV procainamide 10 mg/kg body weight over 5 minutes.

If Rhythm Is Broad and Irregular

　　　Do *not* give digitalis or verapamil.
　　　Give IV procainamide 10 mg/kg body weight IV over 5 minutes.
　　　If unsuccessful, cardiovert (see also Appendix 2).

If Rhythm Is Torsade de Pointes

Transmit the 12-lead ECG to the base hospital.
　　　History will usually implicate class IA or III drugs.
　　　Maintain continuous monitoring.
　　　Establish IV line; physician may advise to begin IV magnesium. IV

magnesium is advocated even in normomagnesemia. Give MgCl or $MgSO_4$ 1 to 2 gm IV bolus over 5 minutes; infusion: 1 to 2 gm/hour for 4 to 6 hours.

If IV magnesium is unsuccessful, advise physician because cardiac pacing may be necessary upon arrival at hospital (see also Chapter 9).

If History Suggests Digitalis Intoxication

Transmit the 12-lead ECG to the base hospital.

Protect the patient from stress (catecholamines may exacerbate the arrhythmia).

Do not use vagal maneuvers.

Establish an IV line and transport without delay.

Continue monitoring.

A temporary pacemaker or digitalis antibodies may be indicated upon arrival at the hospital.

UNCONSCIOUS PATIENT IN TACHYCARDIA

1. Cardiovert; transmit the 12-lead ECG to the base hospital.
2. Obtain vital signs and a history from the family if possible; advise the physician especially concerning medications being taken by the patient.
3. Establish an IV line.

UNCONSCIOUS PATIENT IN BRADYCARDIA

1. Record a 12-lead ECG; transmit to the base hospital.
2. Take a history and do a physical examination.
3. Give IV atropine 0.04 mg/kg body weight.
4. Advise physician of results because temporary pacing may be necessary if atropine is unsuccessful.

CONSCIOUS PATIENT IN BRADYCARDIA

1. Record a 12-lead ECG; transmit to the base hospital.
2. Take a history and do a physical examination.
3. Evaluate the ECG for myocardial infarction, arrhythmia, PR interval, and QRS axis and width.

    Type of arrhythmia: note regularity, abrupt pauses, or group beating. Regularity suggests a sinus bradycardia or heart block; abrupt pauses in the atrial rhythm or group beating suggests SA block or sick sinus syndrome; abrupt pauses or group beating in the ventricular rhythm suggests AV block.

    The PR interval and QRS axis and width will help evaluate for AV and/or intraventricular block.

4. Treatment:

- If sinus bradycardia, give no treatment unless hypotension/hypoperfusion; then administer atropine 0.04 mg/kg body weight.
- If SA block or sinus arrest, give no treatment unless hypotension develops; then give atropine.
- If sick sinus syndrome, advise the physician because a pacemaker may be indicated upon reaching the hospital.
- If complete AV block with narrow QRS, give no treatment unless hypotension/hypoperfusion; then give atropine and advise physician because a pacemaker may be indicated upon reaching the hospital.

If complete AV block with broad QRS, with or without hypotension, a temporary pacemaker may be indicated.

ENERGY SETTINGS FOR DEFIBRILLATION AND FOR CARDIOVERSION OF UNCONSCIOUS PATIENTS

In VT and SVT, administer 10 J (synchronized); if not effective, give 100 J.

In ventricular fibrillation, give 200 J (unsynchronized); if not effective, use 350 J. In children 2.5 to 50 kg, defibrillate with 2 J/kg.

References

1. Karagounis, L., Ipsen, S.K., Jessop, M.R., et al.: Impact of field-transmitted electrocardiography on time to in-hospital thrombolytic therapy in acute myocardial infarction. Am. J. Cardiol. 66:786–791, 1990.
2. Gunnar, R.M., Bourdillon, P.D.V., Dixon, D.W., et al.: ACC/AHA guidelines for the early management of patients with acute myocardial infarction. Circulation 82:664–707, 1990.

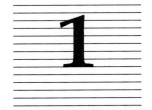

Emergency Axis Determination

RAPID AXIS DETERMINATION

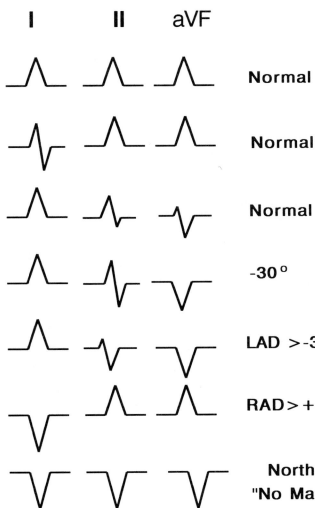

I	II	aVF	
			Normal
			Normal
			Normal
			-30°
			LAD > -30°
			RAD > +120°
			Northwest "No Man's Land"

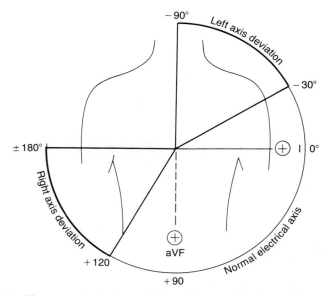

Figure App. 1–1. The normal and abnormal electrical axes of the heart. Normal axis = +120 degrees to −30 degrees; abnormal left axis > −30 degrees; abnormal right axis > +120 degrees.

THE NORMAL QRS AXIS

The QRS axis is the sum of all the currents generated within the ventricles during electrical systole (mean current flow); it is usually to the left and inferior, but may be anywhere between the left shoulder (−30 degrees) and the right hip (+120 degrees) and still be normal (Fig. App. 1–1).

CLINICAL USE OF AXIS DETERMINATION

QRS AXIS

QRS axis determination is of importance in the emergency situations of:

1. *Acute myocardial infarction* (to diagnose hemiblock and identify high-risk patients). In anterior (superior) hemiblock there is an abnormal left axis deviation (ALAD) of greater than −30 degrees; in posterior (inferior) hemiblock there is right axis deviation (RAD) of greater than +120 degrees.
2. *Acute pulmonary embolism,* where there is often a shift in the QRS axis to the right.
3. *Wide QRS tachycardia,* where an abnormal axis supports a diagnosis of ventricular tachycardia. An axis in the northwest quadrant is highly suggestive of ventricular tachycardia. In lead V_1-positive wide QRS tachycardia, an abnormal axis (left or right) supports a diagnosis of ventricular tachycardia. In lead V_1-negative wide QRS tachycardia, a right axis deviation is diagnostic of ventricular tachycardia.

BEST LEAD COMBINATIONS FOR RAPID AXIS DETERMINATION

Rapid axis determination can be made using leads I and II or I and aVF, or by the "easy two-step" method. The normal axis is between −30 degrees and +120 degrees;

left axis deviation (LAD) is greater than -30 degrees; RAD is greater than $+120$ degrees.

Of the three rapid methods of axis determination, the combination of leads I and II is the most useful, being very sensitive to axis shifts to the left and within the left quadrant. Use of the combination of leads I and aVF has disadvantages in the setting of acute anterior wall myocardial infarction and requires the addition of a third lead. The easy two-step is more accurate but is not as fast as the other two methods. The advantages and disadvantages are discussed below.

QRS AXIS DETERMINATION USING LEADS I AND II

The fastest method of determining axis is simply to know the QRS combinations in leads I and II, as illustrated at the beginning of this appendix. A glance at these two leads is sufficient in emergency settings, lead II being very sensitive to axis shifts to the left and within the left quadrant.

Normal. Leads I and II are upright (i.e., the sum of the components of each is zero or positive).

Abnormal Left (More Than -30 Degrees). Lead I is positive and lead II is negative (i.e., the sum of its components is negative).

Abnormal Right. Lead I is negative and lead II is positive.

Northwest. Both lead I and lead II are usually negative, although lead II can be negative for an axis deviation to the right of $+150$ degrees as well. (For this quadrant leads I and aVF are better.)

When evaluating the QRS combinations in the illustration at the beginning of this appendix, note the sensitivity of lead II in tracking the axis in the left quadrant. For example,

1. When the axis is within the left quadrant, lead I remains upright, being mostly positive when the mean current is parallel to the axis of lead I (0 degrees) and becoming equiphasic when current flow is perpendicular to the axis of lead I (-90 degrees).
2. Within the left quadrant, the borderline between normal and abnormal is -30 degrees, at which point lead II becomes equiphasic. Thus, when the axis is between 0 and -30 degrees, lead I will be positive, and lead II will be become less and less positive as the axis shifts left; it will become equiphasic when the axis reaches -30 degrees.
3. When the QRS axis is to the left of -30 degrees, lead II will become negative (i.e., the sum of its components is negative), indicating an abnormal left axis deviation.

QRS AXIS DETERMINATION USING LEADS I AND aVF

Normal. Leads I and aVF are positive (i.e., the sum of the components of each is positive).

Left Quadrant. Lead I is positive and lead aVF is negative.

Right Quadrant. Lead I is negative and lead aVF is positive.

Northwest Quadrant. Leads I and aVF are both negative.

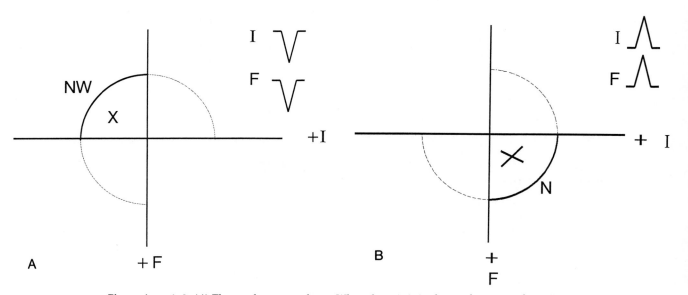

Figure App. 1–2. (*A*) The northwest quadrant. When the axis is in the northwest quadrant ("no man's land"), leads I and aVF are negative. (*B*) The normal quadrant. When the axis is in the normal quadrant, leads I and aVF are positive.

Figure App. 1–2 illustrates that the combination of leads I and aVF is useful in the determination of an axis in the normal quadrant (+90 degrees to 0 degrees) and in the northwest quadrant (−90 degrees to ±180 degrees). However, this combination of leads does not differentiate between normal left and abnormal left when the axis is within the left quadrant. For example, if lead I is positive and lead aVF negative, the QRS axis can be anywhere in the left quadrant (0 degrees to −90 degrees), as illustrated in Figure App. 1–3. Since part of the left quadrant is within normal range, this is not a useful observation in the setting of acute anterior wall myocardial infarction. In this setting, a shift in the axis to the left of −30 degrees identifies a

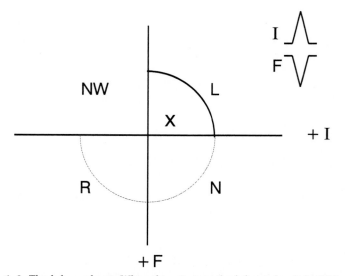

Figure App. 1–3. The left quadrant. When the axis is in the left quadrant, lead I is positive and lead aVF is negative. However, the axis is not considered to be abnormal until it is to the left of −30 degrees, a fact that is not possible to determine using leads I and aVF alone.

patient with superior (left anterior) hemiblock, whereas a left axis of 0 to −30 degrees would not be considered diagnostic of such a condition.

Thus, when using leads I and aVF for axis determination, an additional lead is necessary to determine in which part of the left quadrant the axis lies.

QRS AXIS DETERMINATION BY THE EASY TWO-STEP

The next fastest method of axis determination involves the use of two of the six limb leads: the one in which the QRS is equiphasic or is almost so, and the one that is parallel to that current. For this you must know where the six limb leads are and understand Einthoven's triangle, unipolar limb leads, and the orientation of mean current flow to lead axis.

EINTHOVEN'S TRIANGLE

Willem Einthoven introduced the three bipolar limb leads that define Einthoven's triangle, shown in Figure App. 1–4. It is composed of leads I, II, and III; these are the only bipolar leads in the 12-lead ECG. Lead I is across the shoulders with the negative electrode on the right shoulder and the positive electrode on the left shoulder; lead II is on the right side of the body with the negative electrode also on the right shoulder and the positive electrode at the apex of the triangle; lead III is on the left side of the body with the negative electrode on the left shoulder and the positive electrode at the apex of the triangle.

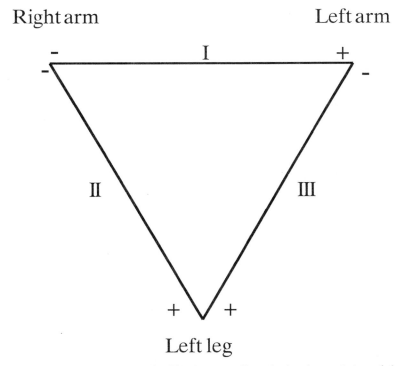

Figure App. 1–4. Einthoven's triangle. This is an equilateral triangle consisting of the three bipolar limb leads—I, II, and III. Lead I creates an electrical potential between the arms, and leads II and III create an electrical potential between the arms and the left leg.

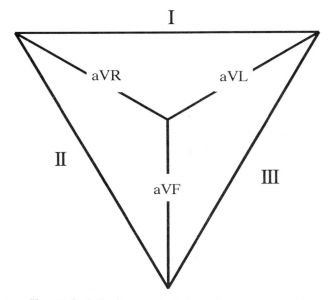

Figure App. 1–5. The six limb leads consist of Einthoven's equilateral triangle plus three unipolar leads. The unipolar limb leads are achieved by placing a positive electrode on each arm (aVR and aVL) and one on the left leg (aVF). There is an electrical potential between this positive electrode and a reference point at the center of Einthoven's triangle.

UNIPOLAR LIMB LEADS

The unipolar limb leads are formed by a positive electrode at each point of Einthoven's triangle and the zero reference point in the center of the electrical field of the heart. This reference point is created by the sum of the electrical potentials from the three bipolar leads. The lead axes of the three unipolar and three bipolar limb leads are illustrated in Figure App. 1–5.

THE HEXAXIAL FIGURE

The hexaxial figure provides an excellent reference system for estimating the axis in degrees. This figure is drawn by shifting the axes of the six limb leads so that they all pass through the center of the heart's electrical field (Fig. App. 1–6).

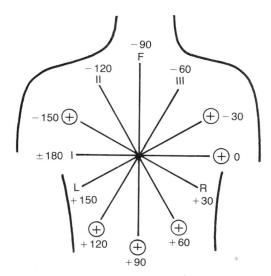

Figure App. 1–6. The hexaxial figure. All lead axes are drawn through the center of the electrical field of the heart; each lead axis has a 30-degree angle with its neighboring lead axis.

ORIENTATION OF CURRENT FLOW TO THE LEAD AXIS

When the mean current of the heart is perpendicular to the axis of a lead, an equiphasic deflection is produced. When this current is parallel with the axis of the lead, the resulting ECG complex is either the most positive or the most negative deflection, depending upon whether current flows toward the positive or the negative electrode.

FIGURING THE AXIS

Step 1. Find the equiphasic deflection; the mean current of the heart is perpendicular to this lead axis. If there is no equiphasic deflection in any of the six limb leads, choose the one that is smallest (i.e., almost equiphasic). In order to discover in which direction this current is traveling, proceed to the next step.

Step 2. Now look at the QRS complex in the lead with an axis parallel to the current flow. For example, if the equiphasic deflection were in lead III as in Figure App. 1–7, the mean current would be perpendicular to the axis of lead III and parallel to the axis of lead aVR. Thus, if lead aVR is negative, as shown in Figure App. 1–7, the axis is normal.

PRACTICAL APPLICATIONS

The 12-lead ECGs in Figures App. 1–8 to 1–10 are from patients seen in the setting of acute anterior wall MI, broad QRS tachycardia, and pulmonary embolism. The axis determination was important in the definitive diagnosis. The answers are in the legends, but before reading them, determine each axis for yourself.

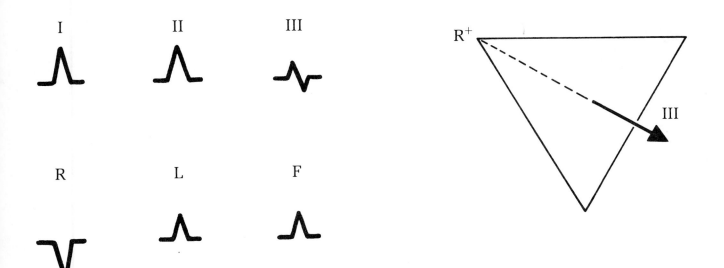

Figure App. 1–7. The equiphasic complex in lead III indicates that the mean current is perpendicular to the axis of lead III. Lead aVR reveals which way this current is flowing, because the axis of aVR is parallel with the current flow.

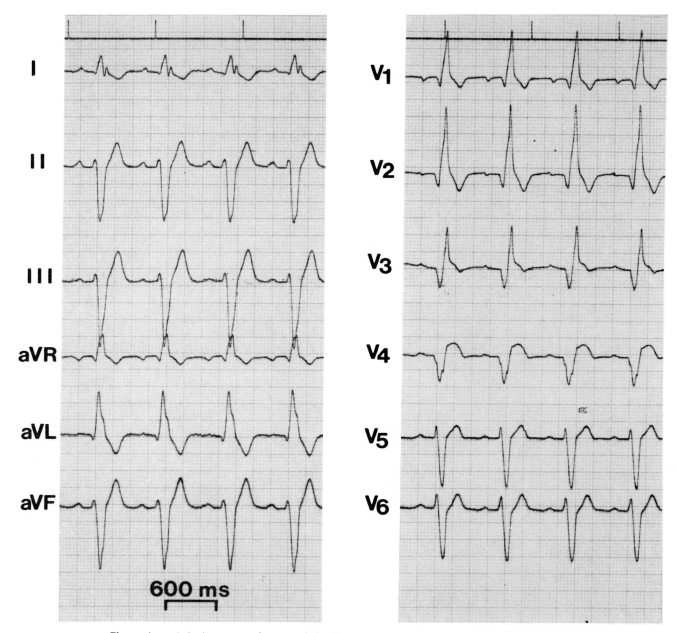

Figure App. 1–8. Anteroseptal myocardial infarction with right bundle branch block. The left axis deviation reflects left anterior hemiblock and indicates more extensive myocardial damage. That finding classifies the patient as being at risk for pump failure and severe ventricular arrhythmias and calls for an aggressive therapeutic approach.

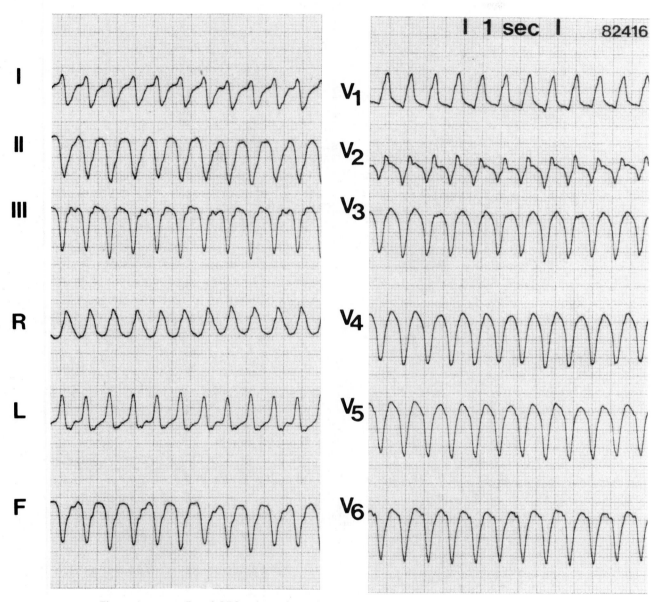

Figure App. 1–9. Broad QRS tachycardia with an axis in the northwest quadrant (down in leads I, II, III). Such an axis is diagnostic of VT. (See also Chapter 8.)

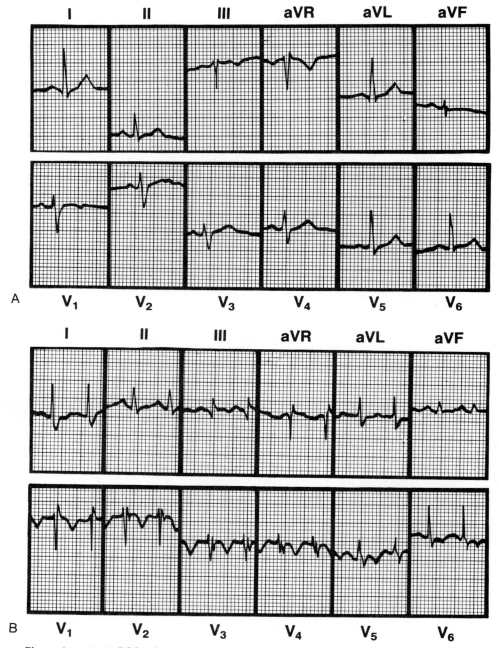

Figure App. 1–10. ECGs after pulmonary embolism. Following the sudden onset of chest pain, the sinus rate accelerates (sinus tachycardia), the axis shifts to the right (from 0 degrees in the top tracing to +45 degrees in the bottom tracing), and right-sided conduction delay develops. (Note the appearance of a late R wave in lead V_1.)

P WAVE AXIS DETERMINATION

CLINICAL USE

P wave axis determination is useful in the differential diagnosis of supraventricular tachycardia and in acute pulmonary embolism. For example, a negative P wave in lead I during paroxysmal supraventricular tachycardia indicates that a left-sided accessory pathway is being used as the retrograde arm of a reentry circuit. This is discussed in more detail in Chapter 4.

Slight axis shifts during sinus rhythm may represent normal shifts in pacing sites within the SA node.

METHOD OF DETERMINING P AXIS

The P wave axis is determined in the same way as the QRS axis. In the six limb leads, look for the smallest P wave; if it is isoelectric, the mean P vector is perpendicular to that lead axis. Next, look at the P wave in the lead with an axis parallel to the current flow. A positive P wave indicates that the mean current flow is toward the positive electrode of that lead, just as when figuring the QRS axis. If the smallest P wave was not precisely isoelectric, an adjustment can now be made, since the P vector could not then be exactly perpendicular.

SUMMARY

QRS axis determination is useful in the emergency settings of acute myocardial infarction, acute pulmonary embolism, and wide complex tachycardia.

Instant recognition is achieved by observing the polarity of the complexes in leads I and II or in leads I and aVF. When there is more time or when a finer degree of accuracy is desired, the axis can be plotted in the hexaxial figure.

Using the combination of leads I and II, in the normal axis these leads are positive (i.e., the sum of the components in each of the leads is positive) in leads I and II; abnormal left axis is positive in lead I and negative in lead II; abnormal right axis is negative in lead I and positive in lead aVF. The advantage of this method is that it is very sensitive to shifts of axis within the left quadrant; its disadvantage is that it does not pinpoint an axis within the northwest quadrant.

The combination of leads I and aVF defines the quadrant that the axis occupies. The axis is in the normal quadrant when the complexes in leads I and aVF are positive. The axis is in the left quadrant when lead I is positive and lead aVF is negative. The axis is in the right quadrant when lead I is negative and lead aVF is positive. The axis is in the northwest quadrant when both leads I and aVF are negative. The advantage of this combination of leads is that it accurately and rapidly determines an axis in the northwest quadrant; its disadvantage is that it does not differentiate between a normal and an abnormal left axis without the use of a third lead.

APPENDIX

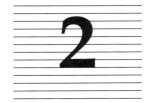

2

Electrical Treatment of Arrhythmias

CARDIOVERSION AND DEFIBRILLATION

Cardioversion is the electrical conversion of an atrial or ventricular arrhythmia to a normal sinus rhythm. This is accomplished by the delivery of a direct current (DC) shock to the heart. The current is synchronized to discharge with the QRS complex. During tachycardia, the electrical current depolarizes the heart and interrupts the arrhythmia; during fibrillation, the current reduces the amount of excitable myocardium so that fibrillation cannot be perpetuated. Synchronization of the electrical discharge with the QRS complex is necessary to avoid delivering a depolarizing current during the "vulnerable period" when the heart is more susceptible to ventricular fibrillation. The "vulnerable period" is an interval that begins and ends with the T wave but that is at its peak for about 30 msec just before the apex of the T wave. At this point, the current required to elicit ventricular fibrillation is at its lowest. Additionally, in the ischemic heart the stimulus required to cause fibrillation is much less than it is in the normal heart.

EMERGENCY CARDIOVERSION

Cardioversion is performed promptly with minimal premedication on patients who have tachycardia and discernible R and T waves and a deteriorating hemodynamic status. This would include those with

1. Atrial flutter or atrial fibrillation with conduction over an accessory pathway that does not respond to procainamide or ajmaline (in Europe) or is associated with hemodynamic instability
2. Supraventricular tachycardia that does not respond to vagal maneuvers or antiarrhythmic therapy, is not caused by digitalis intoxication, and is associated with hemodynamic instability
3. Ventricular tachycardia that is refractory to antiarrhythmic drug therapy and is associated with hemodynamic instability

DEFIBRILLATION

Defibrillation is nonsynchronized cardioversion; it is used when QRS complexes and T waves are not distinguishable, as in ventricular fibrillation. Early defibrillation is the most useful measure in resuscitation; the earlier it is initiated, the better the chance of success. Even if the rhythm appears to be asystole, it may still respond to defibrillation because, depending upon the recorded ECG lead, both fine and coarse ventricular fibrillation may mimic asystole. The coarse fibrillation waves of ventricular fibrillation may actually produce zero electrical vectors, resulting in a relatively straight line.[1, 2]

RISKS

Risks associated with cardioversion and defibrillation include:

Postcardioversion tachyarrhythmias (ventricular tachycardia or ventricular fibrillation)
Bradyarrhythmias or asystole
Embolism (systemic or pulmonary)
Myocardial injury
Ventricular dysfunction
Pulmonary edema
Hypotension

CHOICE OF ENERGY SETTING

Ventricular Tachycardia. Ten joules (10 J) is usually adequate; 100 J is almost always effective.

Atrial Flutter. Begin with 20 J; energy levels that are too low (5–10 J) may convert atrial flutter to atrial fibrillation. If 20 J is not effective, use 50 or 100 J on repeat attempt.

Supraventricular Tachycardia. Ten joules (10 J) is frequently effective, whereas 100 J is almost always successful.

Atrial Fibrillation. Initial suggested shock strength is 100 J. If not successful, a higher energy shock (200 or 300 J) may be delivered.

Ventricular Fibrillation. Initially 200 J; if unsuccessful this is followed immediately by 350 J. (For children weighing 2.5–50 kg, use 2 J/kg.)

Digitalis Toxicity. In cases of possible or suspected digitalis excess or subclinical digitalis toxicity, it may be safer to start all electrical cardioversion at 5 to 10 J. This may be enough to restore normal sinus rhythm, except in atrial fibrillation, in which case this "test dose" may disclose warning ventricular arrhythmias secondary to subclinical digitalis excess. In this situation the procedure is best terminated and alternative antiarrhythmic therapy planned.

CARDIOVERSION FOR PATIENTS WITH IMPLANTED PACEMAKERS

Patients with implanted pacing systems needing emergency cardioversion or defibrillation require special attention to avoid endocardial burns and/or increased fibrosis at the electrode-endocardial interface. Energy can be shunted to the myocardium via the pacing electrode, causing endocardial burns and an increase in the stimulation threshold; this in turn results in a loss of capture.[3]

Infrequently, damage to the pulse generator may occur if the energy transmitted by the cardioverter exceeds the level of protection built into the device. This may render the unit nonfunctional or change its mode and program of pacing.

The following precautions should therefore be taken when the patient has a pacemaker:

1. Position the defibrillator paddles at least 13 cm away from the pulse generator. This may necessitate anterior-posterior or apical-posterior paddle placement. If anterior-posterior paddles are not available, keep the paddle as far from the pulse generator as possible and use the lowest effective energy level.
2. Have the pacemaker programmer available so that the pacemaker output can be reprogrammed immediately in case of loss of capture.
3. Within hours and periodically for the next two months following the shock, check for a rise in stimulation threshold. If there is a rise in the stimulation threshold, a concomitant increase in the delivered energy from the pulse generator will be necessary. This may result in a shortening of the life of the system, and careful followup is indicated.
4. If the patient is clearly pacemaker dependent, consider the addition of a temporary backup pacemaker prior to elective cardioversion.
5. Most external pacers can stand electrical shocks of 400 J. For additional safety, turn off the pacemaker pulse generator before defibrillation.

PRECORDIAL THUMP

Rapid hypotensive ventricular tachycardia can sometimes be converted to a supraventricular rhythm by a forceful blow to the sternum with the fleshy part of the fist; this may be repeated once. Such a blow, properly administered, may deliver a low-level electrical shock (approximately 5 mV) to the heart.

Disadvantages are possible conversion of ventricular tachycardia into ventricular fibrillation or into a faster ventricular tachycardia, further hemodynamic deterioration, and wasted time and effort in a situation where seconds count. The American Heart Association recommends the thump version only for monitored cardiac arrest with ventricular tachycardia when electrical defibrillation is immediately available.

EMERGENCY TREATMENT OF POSTCARDIOVERSION ARRHYTHMIAS

Cardioversion may be followed by bradyarrhythmia or asystole, especially if there is pre-existing AV block or sick sinus syndrome. Emergency treatment includes IV atropine, isoproterenol (Isuprel), or a temporary pacemaker. Postconversion ventricular tachycardia and ventricular fibrillation are rare and almost always the result of incorrect synchronization; treat with nonsynchronized DC defibrillation. Lidocaine (in the acute ischemic setting), procainamide (when an acute ischemic attack can be ruled out), or bretylium may be needed for treatment of recurrent ventricular tachycardia or ventricular fibrillation.

In cases where ventricular tachycardia or ventricular fibrillation is secondary to digitalis toxicity (Chapter 8), a temporary pacemaker, phenytoin (Dilantin 250 mg IV over 5 minutes), digitalis antibody (Digibind), or IV magnesium sulfate or magnesium chloride (2 gm IV over 1–2 minutes) may be required.

EMERGENCY PACING

Emergency pacing is rarely needed during cardiopulmonary resuscitation. Ventricular fibrillation is treated with defibrillation and drugs. Electromechanical dissociation is frequently based upon inadequate coronary perfusion or myocardial rupture with pericardial tamponade and does not respond to pacing. In bradyasystolic cardiac arrest, apart from airway establishment with effective ventilation and institution of chest compression and the use of drugs (epinephrine, atropine), emergency pacing may be required.

References

1. Ewy, G. A.: Recent advances in cardiopulmonary resuscitation and defibrillation. Curr. Probl. Cardiol. 8(1):5–42, 1983.
2. Weaver, W. K., Cobb, L. A., Dennis, D., et al.: Amplitude of ventricular fibrillation waveform and outcome after cardiac arrest. Ann. Intern. Med. 102:53–55, 1985.
3. Gould, L., Patel, S., Gomes, G. I., et al.: Pacemaker failure following external defibrillation. PACE 4:575–577, 1981.

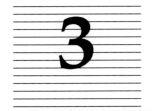

3

Emergency Drugs

Table App. 3–1. **Intravenous Dosage (Adult) of Drugs Commonly Used During Bradycardia, Tachycardia, or Following Cardiopulmonary Resuscitation***

Drug	Dosage
Adenosine (Adenocard)	6–12 mg
Atropine	0.5–1.0 mg
Bretylium (Bretylol)	2–5 mg/kg
Calcium chloride	500 mg or 6.8 mEq (5 ml of 10% solution)
Digoxin (Lanoxin)	0.125–0.5 mg
Ephedrine	5–10 mg
Epinephrine (Adrenalin)	0.5–1.0 mg
Lidocaine (Xylocaine)	1–1.5 mg/kg bodyweight
Magnesium sulfate or magnesium chloride	1–2 gm (5–10 ml of 20% solution)
Nitroglycerin (Tridil)	200 –400 μg
Phenytoin (Dilantin)	100–250 mg IV at 50 mg/min†
Procainamide (Pronestyl)	10 mg/kg/min to 1000 mg
Propranolol (Inderal)	1–2 mg
Sodium bicarbonate	1 mEq/kg
	50–75 ml of 8.4% solution
Verapamil (Isoptin, Calan)	5–10 mg in 2–3 min

*Usually mixed in 5–10 ml D5W or normal saline.
†Use 0.22–0.45 micron filter.

Table App. 3–2. **Infusion Mixtures for Drugs Used During Bradycardia, Tachycardia, or Following Cardiopulmonary Resuscitation**

Drug	Dose Concentration Per 250 ml D5W	Usual Dose Per ml	Per minute*
Bretylium (Bretylol)	1000 mg	4 mg	1–2 mg
Dobutamine (Dobutrex)	500 mg	2 mg	5–15 μg/kg
Dopamine (Inotropin)	200 mg	800 μg	2.5–20 μg/kg†
Epinephrine (Adrenalin)	1 mg	4 μg	1–8 μg
Isoproterenol (Isuprel)	2 mg	8 μg	1–8 μg
Lidocaine (Xylocaine)	1000 mg	4 mg	1–4 mg
Magnesium sulfate	4 gm	16 mg	16 mg
Nitroglycerin (Tridil, Nitrostat, Nitro-Bid, Nitrocine, Nitrol)	50 mg	200 μg	25–1000 μg
Nitroprusside (Nipride, Nitropress)	50 mg	200 μg	10–500 μg
Norepinephrine (Levophed)	4 mg	16 μg	1–8 μg
Phenytoin (Dilantin)	500 mg	2 mg	200–300 μg
Procainamide (Pronestyl)	1000 mg	4 mg	1–4 mg

*Usually started at a low dose and titrated to desired action. If high doses are used, use higher concentration (×2, ×4) to limit volume of infusion.

†Low dose: 2.5 to 5 μg/kg/min. High dose: (predominant alpha action) 5 to 20 μg/kg/min. For high dose infusion, use a more concentrated solution.

Table App. 3–3. **Dosage of Drugs Used Intravenously for Treatment During Circus Movement Tachycardia Using an Accessory Pathway**

Adenosine 6 mg; if unsuccessful 12 mg and may repeat
Verapamil 10 mg over 3 min
Ajmaline 1 mg/kg over 3 min
Procainamide 10 mg/kg over 5 min
Diltiazem hydrochloride 0.25 mg/kg

Table App. 3–4. **Dosage of Drugs Used Intravenously for Treatment During Atrial Fibrillation in Patients Using an Accessory Pathway**

Procainamide 10 mg/kg over 5 min
Ajmaline 1 mg/kg over 3 min
Disopyramide 1.5 to 2 mg/kg over 5 min

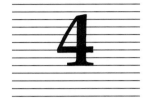

Minimal Emergency Diagnostic Leads

It is highly recommended and advantageous to record 12-lead ECGs in all patients with rhythm disturbances. However, because of equipment limitations in many critical care units and emergency rooms, we are aware that this is not always possible. It may not even be possible to secure a 12-lead ECG while the tachycardia is in progress. We have therefore included comments in the text and a table here to guide you in your selection of leads, depending on the clinical setting. The leads listed here are absolute minimal requirements for a diagnosis; you cannot do less.

When only two electrodes are available, as may be the case in some telemetry units, the electrodes should be applied and then unsnapped and snapped into position until the necessary number of leads are collected. To record a simulated V lead, place the negative electrode under the left clavicle and the positive electrode in the desired precordial position for MCL1 (V_1), MCL2 (V_2), and MCL6 (V_6) (Fig. App. 4–1).

In cases of paroxysmal supraventricular tachycardia, the patient should be instructed not to terminate the tachycardia (by coughing and so forth) until the

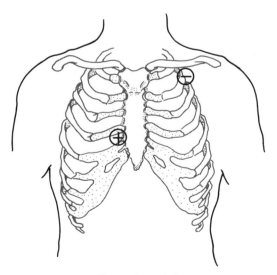

Figure App. 4–1

rhythm has been recorded in multiple leads (at least leads I, II, III, V_1, and V_6). The sinus rhythm must then be recorded in the same leads so that a comparison can be made that may reveal the position of the P waves.

Table App. 4–1. **Diagnostic Leads***

Digitalis Toxicity	Supraventricular Tachycardia	Wide QRS Tachycardia	Unstable Angina
Atrial activity: Lead II for P waves *Fascicular VT:* Lead V_1 for right bundle branch block; leads I and II for axis	Leads I, II, III, V_1, and V_6 to locate P waves; compare tachycardia with sinus rhythm in these leads.	For V_1-negative: Leads V_1, V_2, and V_6; for V_1-positive: Leads V_1 and V_6	Lead V_2 when without pain; 12-lead ECG when with pain
See Chapter 8	See Chapter 4	See Chapter 3	See Chapter 2

*See specific chapters listed here for further explanation.

Index

Note: Page numbers in *italics* refer to illustrations; page numbers followed by (t) refer to tables.

Circus movement tachycardia (Continued)
slowly conducting accessory pathway in, 81, 87–89, 88, 89, 89(t)
anatomical substrate of, 87
ECG recognition of, 87–88, 89, 89(t)
mechanism of, 87, 88
P wave in, 88, 89, 89(t), 90(t), 91
pacemaker-mediated, 182–184, 183
vagal stimulation in, 97–98
Coronary artery, anatomy of, 13–14, 14
left anterior descending (LAD) branch of, stenosis of, prehospital, 193
unstable angina and, 30–32, 31, 32
main, left, ECG recognition of, 192
occlusion of, in inferior myocardial infarction, 7, 7, 8
Coronary artery disease, ventricular bigeminy in, 153
Coughing, 98

Defibrillation, energy setting for, 212
in unconscious patient, 197
indications for, 211–212
pacemaker damage and, 212–213
risks of, 212
Delta wave, in supraventricular tachycardia, 63
Dialysis, in severe hyperkalemia, 173
Digitalis, block sites with, 168(t)
dosage of, amiodarone and, 142, 142(t)
diltiazem and, 142(t), 143
quinidine and, 142, 142(t)
verapamil and, 142(t), 143
dosage requirements in, 142(t), 142–143
serum level of, 156
sinoatrial block and, 167
sinus bradycardia and, 106
Digitalis intoxication, QRS segment in, 54
Digitalis toxicity, 139–159
atrial fibrillation in, 145–146, 147, 148, 157, 158(t)
atrial flutter in, 146, 150, 158, 158(t)
atrial tachycardia in, with block, 143–145, 144
atrioventricular junctional tachycardia in, 145, 146, 158(t)
atrioventricular nodal block and, 167
atrioventricular nodal Wenckebach conduction in, 155
bidirectional ventricular tachycardia in, 153, 154
cardioversion in, 212
carotid sinus massage in, 157
delayed afterdepolarization in, 140, 141
diagnostic approach to, 139
double tachycardia in, 152
drug interactions in, 142(t), 142–143
ECG recognition of, 143–155, 144, 146–152, 154–156, 157–158, 158(t)
leads for, 218(t)
emergency management of, 139

Digitalis toxicity (Continued)
fascicular ventricular tachycardia in, 150–153, 151, 152, 158(t)
axis deviation in, 153
QRS duration in, 153
right bundle branch block pattern in, 150, 151
mechanism of, 140–141, 141
mortality in, 141
non-ECG signs of, 156
P wave in, 144, 145, 158(t)
pacing in, 157
patient history in, 156
prehospital, treatment of, 196
right bundle branch block in, 150, 151
sinoatrial block in, 153, 155, 156
sinus bradycardia in, 153, 155
systematic evaluation of, 157–158, 158(t)
treatment of, 156–157
ventricular bigeminy in, 153, 155
ventriculophasic PP intervals in, 144, 145
Digoxin (Lanoxin), 215(t)
Dilantin (phenytoin), 215(t), 216(t)
Diltiazem, 216(t)
atrioventricular nodal block and, 167
block sites with, 168(t)
digitalis dosage and, 142(t), 143
Disopyramide, 216(t)
block sites with, 168(t)
digitalis dosage and, 143
sinoatrial block and, 167, 168(t)
ventricular arrhythmia with, 163
Dive reflex, 98
Dobutamine (Dobutrex), 216(t)
Dopamine (Inotropin), 216(t)
Drug(s), antiarrhythmic, proarrhythmic effects of, 161–168. See also Bradycardia, drug-induced; Torsades de pointes; Ventricular tachycardia, drug-induced.
digitalis dosage adjustment and, 142(t), 143
IC class, ventricular tachycardia and, 166, 166
second-degree sinoatrial block and, 108
sick sinus syndrome and, 112
sinus arrest and, 108
sinus bradycardia and, 106

Echo beat, in ventricular tachycardia, 57, 59
Einthoven's triangle, in QRS axis determination, 203, 203
Electrical alternans. See QRS alternans.
Electromyographic inhibition, in pacing, 186–187, 187
Embolism, pulmonary, 129–138. See also Pulmonary embolism.
Encainide, block sites with, 168(t)
reentry mechanism with, 162
sinoatrial block and, 167
ventricular tachycardia and, 166

Ephedrine, 215(t)
Epinephrine (Adrenalin), 215(t), 216(t)
Ethmozine, digitalis dosage and, 143
Exercise, in atrioventricular block determination, 116(t)
Eyeball, pressure to, 98

Fascicular ventricular tachycardia, digitalis toxicity and, 150–153, *151, 152,* 158(t)
Fibrillation, atrial. See *Atrial fibrillation.*
  ventricular, 212
Flecainide, block sites with, 168(t)
  digitalis dosage and, 143
  reentry mechanism with, 162
  sinoatrial block and, 167
  ventricular tachycardia and, 166
Frog sign, in narrow QRS tachycardia, 76, 76(t)
Fusion beat, in ventricular tachycardia, 57, *58*

Gagging, 98
Glucose, in severe hyperkalemia, 173

Heart, clockwise rotation of, in acute pulmonary embolism, 132, *132*
Heart sound, first, in atrioventricular dissociation, 40
  in narrow QRS tachycardia, 76(t)
  in supraventricular tachycardia, 75
Hemiblock, 15–16, 16(t)
  anterior, left, acute myocardial infarction and, 22–23, *23*
    ECG recognition of, 22, *23*
    mechanism of, 22–23
  posterior, left, acute myocardial infarction and, 23–25, *24*
    ECG recognition of, *24,* 25
    mechanism of, 25
Hemodialysis, in severe hyperkalemia, 173
Hexaxial figure, in QRS axis determination, 204, *204*
His bundle, 13, *14*
His bundle electrogram, in atrioventricular block determination, *116,* 117
His-Purkinje block, drug-induced, 167, 168(t)
Hyperkalemia, 170–173, *171–173*
  ECG changes in, 170, *171*
  emergency approach to, 169
  mechanism of, 170
  mild, 171
    treatment of, 172
  progressive, 170, *171*
  severe, 170, *171–173*
    treatment of, 172–173, *173*

Hypertension, ventricular, right, in pulmonary embolism, 137–138
Hypokalemia, *174,* 174–176, *175*
  ECG changes in, 174, *174, 175,* 176
  emergency approach to, 169–170
  mechanism of, 174
  progressive, 174, *174, 175,* 176
  T wave in, 174, *174,* 176
  treatment of, 176
  U wave in, 174, *174, 175,* 176
Hypotension, sinus bradycardia and, 106

Idioventricular rhythm, accelerated, in acute myocardial infarction, 10–11, *12*
  QRS configuration of, 11
"Incessant" circus movement tachycardia, 87–89. See also *Circus movement tachycardia, orthodromic, slowly conducting accessory pathway in.*
Indecainide, ventricular tachycardia and, 166
Inderal (propranolol), 215(t)
  sinus bradycardia and, 167
Infarction. See *Myocardial infarction.*
Inotropin (dopamine), 216(t)
Ischemia, nontransmural, 31
  subendocardial, 31
Isoproterenol (Isuprel), 216(t)
Isoptin. See *Verapamil (Calan, Isoptin).*

Jugular pulse, in ventricular tachycardia, 40

LAD stenosis, prehospital, 193
  unstable angina and, 30–32, *31, 32*
Lanoxin (digoxin), 215(t)
Lead(s), 217–218, 218(t)
  aVF, in QRS axis determination, 201–203, *202*
  for rapid axis determinations, 200–201
  I, in QRS axis determination, *199,* 201–203, *202*
  II, in QRS axis determination, *199,* 201
  in digitalis toxicity, 218(t)
  in supraventricular tachycardia, 218(t)
  in unstable angina, 218(t)
  in wide QRS tachycardia, 46–47, 218(t)
  V₁, in ventricular tachycardia, 49, *51,* 51–54, *53*
    in wide QRS tachycardia, 194
  V₄R, in acute myocardial infarction, 192
    in inferior acute myocardial infarction, 6–10, *7–10*
      ST segment of, circumflex artery occlusion and, 7, *7*
        coronary artery occlusion and, 7, *7*

Wide QRS Tachycardia

EMERGENCY APPROACH

Do not panic when confronted with the broad QRS tachycardia. Obtain a 12-lead ECG.

IF HEMODYNAMICALLY UNSTABLE

1. Cardiovert.
2. Obtain a history.
3. Examine the pre- and postcardioversion ECGs to determine the etiology of the arrhythmia.

IF HEMODYNAMICALLY STABLE

1. Examine the patient for clinical signs of AV dissociation.
2. Systematically evaluate the 12-lead ECG.
3. Obtain a history.

IF VENTRICULAR TACHYCARDIA

1. Give procainamide 10 mg/kg body weight IV over 5 minutes unless the tachycardia is ischemia-related; then give lidocaine. If unsuccessful:

over

Narrow QRS Tachycardia

EMERGENCY APPROACH

Obtain a 12-lead ECG.
Assess the hemodynamic situation.

IF HEMODYNAMICALLY UNSTABLE

1. Cardiovert.
2. Obtain a history.
3. Record postconversion ECG.
4. Examine and compare pre- and postcardioversion ECGs to determine the type of supraventricular tachycardia, using a systematic approach.

IF HEMODYNAMICALLY STABLE

1. Look for the "frog sign" in the jugular pulse.
2. Perform vagal stimulation; if unsuccessful:
3. Give adenosine or verapamil:
   - *Adenosine* 6 mg as a rapid IV bolus; if unsuccessful increase dosage to 12 mg; this may be repeated.
   - *Verapamil* 10 mg IV over 3 minutes; reduce to 5 mg if the patient is taking a beta blocker or is hypotensive; if unsuccessful:

over

Acute Myocardial Infarction

EMERGENCY DECISIONS

1. Ascertain the time from onset of pain.
2. Evaluate 12-lead ECG for:
   Type of myocardial infarction (anterior or inferior)
   ST segment elevation score
   Q waves
   Bundle branch block and hemiblock to identify patients at high risk of dying early; such patients should be managed aggressively.
3. Identify candidates for thrombolytic therapy (ST segment elevation score; how much and in how many leads?).
4. In inferior wall myocardial infarction, record lead V_4R.

ECG Identification of High-Risk Patients With Unstable Angina

EMERGENCY APPROACH

ECG RECOGNITION OF CRITICAL PROXIMAL LEFT ANTERIOR DESCENDING CORONARY ARTERY STENOSIS IN PATIENTS WITH UNSTABLE ANGINA

- Unstable angina
- No elevation or minimally elevated enzymes
- No pathological precordial Q waves
- ST segment in precordial leads (especially V_2, V_3) isoelectric or slightly elevated (1 mm), concave or straight
- Progressive, symmetrical T wave inversion
- ECG signs appearing during pain-free interval and disappearing during period of chest pain

ECG RECOGNITION OF LEFT MAINSTEM AND THREE-VESSEL DISEASE IN PATIENTS WITH UNSTABLE ANGINA

- Record 12-lead ECG during chest pain because ECG may be normal during pain-free period

over

2. Cardiovert.
3. Examine the ECG during the ventricular tachycardia and the ECG during sinus rhythm to determine the etiology of the tachycardia.

IF SUPRAVENTRICULAR TACHYCARDIA WITH ABERRATION

1. Vagal stimulation; if unsuccessful:
2. Adenosine 6 mg by rapid IV bolus; if unsuccessful give 12 mg by rapid IV bolus; this dosage may be repeated once. If unavailable:
3. Verapamil 10 mg IV over 3 minutes; reduce to 5 mg if the patient is taking a beta blocker or is hypotensive. If unsuccessful:
4. Procainamide 10 mg/kg body weight IV over 5 minutes; if unsuccessful:
5. Cardiovert.
6. Examine supraventricular tachycardia and postconversion ECGs to determine mechanism.

IF IN DOUBT

Do not give verapamil; give IV procainamide.

IF IRREGULAR

Do not give digitalis or verapamil.
Give IV procainamide unless torsades de pointes is present (see Chapter 9).

4. Give procainamide 10 mg/kg body weight over 5 minutes; if unsuccessful:
5. Perform electrical cardioversion.
6. Obtain a history.
7. Record a postconversion ECG.
8. Examine and compare the pre- and postconversion ECGs to determine the type of supraventricular tachycardia, using a systematic approach.

- ST segment elevation in leads aVR and V_1
- ST segment depression in eight or more leads

Digitalis-Induced Emergencies

SYSTEMATIC DIAGNOSTIC APPROACH

1. Obtain periodic 12-lead ECGs on all patients in your care taking digitalis.
2. Question the patient regarding noncardiac signs of digitalis toxicity and concomitant medication that may interact with digitalis.
3. Know the ECG signs of digitalis dysrhythmias.
4. Look specifically for bradycardia, tachycardia, inappropriate regularity (such as in atrial fibrillation or flutter), or group beating.

EMERGENCY MANAGEMENT

1. Discontinue digitalis.
2. Bedrest (no sympathetic stimulation!)
3. Continuous ECG monitoring
4. If hemodynamically unstable, phenytoin is indicated unless digitalis antibodies are available.

over

Other Drug-Induced Emergencies

EMERGENCY TREATMENT

TORSADE DE POINTES

1. Stop the offending drug.
2. Continue ECG monitoring.
3. Give magnesium as MgCl or MgSO$_4$ 1 to 2 gm IV bolus over 5 minutes; infusion: 1 to 2 gm per hour for 4 to 6 hours.
4. If IV magnesium is unsuccessful, increase heart rate with isoproterenol or by pacing.

SUSTAINED (INCESSANT) MONOMORPHIC VENTRICULAR TACHYCARDIA

1. Stop the offending drug.
2. In case of hemodynamic compromise, give inotropic support with isoproterenol or epinephrine. This will also counteract slowing in conduction velocity induced by class IA or class IC drugs.
3. If ventricular tachycardia persists and is poorly tolerated, pace the atrium at the rate of the ventricular tachycardia. Use an AV interval that will provide maximal contribution of atrial contraction to ventricular filling.

over

Slow Atrial Rhythms

EMERGENCY APPROACH

1. Record a 12-lead ECG.
2. In case of hypotension and other signs of diminished cardiac output, immediately initiate the following supportive measures: Give IV atropine 0.04 mg/kg body weight. If heart rate does not accelerate, temporary pacing is indicated.
3. If hypotension, dizziness, and presyncope are absent, no immediate treatment is required.
4. Evaluate ECG for:
   - Myocardial infarction
   - Mechanism of bradycardia: Note regularity, abrupt pauses, or group beating. P wave regularity indicates a regular sinus or atrial rhythm; abrupt pauses in the sinus rhythm or group beating suggests SA block; abrupt pauses or group beating in the ventricular rhythm suggests AV block.
   - QRS axis and width for coexistent bundle branch block
5. If sinus bradycardia is demonstrated, give no treatment unless hypotension is present (give atropine).

over

ECG Recognition of Acute Pulmonary Embolism

EMERGENCY APPROACH

EXAMINE THE ECG FOR

- Rhythm disturbances
- A shift in the axis to the right in comparison with the ECG prior to the acute event (need not be outside the normal range of +90 to −30 degrees)
- Appearance of a right bundle branch block (RBBB) pattern
- Pseudoinfarction patterns

Sudden changes in the ECG suggesting pulmonary embolism call for an emergency echocardiogram.

THERAPY

- Oxygen
- Analgesics
- Full-dose heparin
- Thrombolytic therapy

over

5. Ventricular pacing is indicated:
- In symptomatic bradycardia
- During treatment with phenytoin because suppression of the tachycardia may be followed by asystole
6. Correct potassium and magnesium deficits.

AVOID
1. Sympathetic stimulation (stress, anxiety, exercise, sympathomimetic drugs)
2. Carotid sinus massage
3. Fast or sudden cessation of pacing

6. In case of SA block or sinus arrest, give no treatment unless hypotension is present or the rhythm is digitalis-induced (stop the drug).
7. If the diagnosis is sick sinus syndrome, treatment will depend upon symptoms (dizziness, presyncope, congestive failure).

DRUG-INDUCED BRADYCARDIA
1. Stop the offending drug.
2. Give atropine or start temporary transvenous pacing in case of (a) Adams-Stokes attacks, (b) a low ventricular rate leading to hypotension, and/or (c) bradycardia-dependent ventricular arrythmias.

PREVENTION
Avoid Venous Stasis
Early mobilization and ambulation when possible
External compression of the legs for patients on complete bedrest.
Anticoagulants
If heart failure is present or the patient is on long-term bedrest

EMERGENCY APPROACH TO HYPO- AND HYPERKALEMIA

ECG RECOGNITION OF SEVERE OR PROGRESSIVE HYPERKALEMIA

- Broad QRS
- Slow heart rate
- Usually left axis deviation
- Loss of P wave
- Loss of ST segment (continuous with S wave)
- Tall tented T wave
- QTc interval normal or shortened

TREATMENT

1. Calcium gluconate (10 percent) 10 to 30 ml IV infusion over 1 to 5 minutes with constant ECG monitoring
2. Hypertonic glucose solution (10 percent) 200 to 500 ml in 30 minutes, and 500 to 1000 ml over the next several hours
3. Sodium bicarbonate (2 to 3 ampuls) may be added to 1 liter of 5 percent dextrose in 0.9 percent saline.

over

EMERGENCY APPROACH

EARLY FAILURE TO CAPTURE AND SENSE

1. If failure to capture, increase the output (amplitude or pulse width).
2. If unsuccessful, reposition the electrode catheter.
3. If failure to sense, increase the sensitivity; when sensing is still inadequate, change to unipolar sensing.
4. If unsuccessful, reposition the catheter.

PACING FAILURE

1. If no pacemaker spikes are present, inspect all conducting wires and connections; record an ECG from each electrode.
2. If there are intermittent pacemaker spikes, only one electrode may be involved; convert to a unipolar system.

PACEMAKER SYNDROME

1. Prevent the pacemaker syndrome by carefully checking for the presence of ventriculoatrial (VA) conduction during temporary pacemaker

over

EMERGENCY APPROACH

2. Decrease atrial sensing sensitivity.
3. Program a short AV interval.
4. Or switch to a DVI mode; this eliminates atrial sensing and terminates the tachycardia.

THROMBOSIS AND PULMONARY EMBOLISM

Heparin and thrombolytic therapy is usually sufficient for clinically important thrombosis.

INFECTION OR EROSION OF THE PULSE GENERATOR

1. A temporary pacemaker is inserted, the entire permanent pacing unit is removed, and a new unit is installed on the contralateral side.
2. The removal of the involved lead is usually difficult, and continuous careful traction is applied to the lead.
3. If this fails, in cases of endocarditis, thoracotomy may be necessary.
4. The lead may be saved in the case of pacemaker erosion if the condition is detected early.

over

ELECTROMYOGRAPHIC INHIBITION (EMI)

1. Decrease the sensitivity of the pacemaker.
2. If unsuccessful, reprogram the pacemaker from a unipolar to a bipolar unit.
3. If unsuccessful, reoperation may be necessary.

EMERGENCY TEMPORARY PACING

Prepare for emergency temporary pacing in the event of:

1. Complete AV block with a slow ventricular escape rhythm
2. Symptomatic sinus bradycardia, asystole, or prolonged sinus pauses
3. Acute anterior myocardial infarction with complete heart block, right bundle branch block (RBBB) or left bundle branch block (LBBB) with type II second-degree AV block or RBBB with new hemiblock
4. Acute inferior myocardial infarction with complete heart block leading to hypotension, congestive heart failure, or ventricular arrhythmias
5. Bradycardia-induced or drug-induced torsade de pointes
6. Malfunction of a permanent pacemaker
7. Digitalis toxicity-induced ventricular tachycardia (VT) being treated with drugs (e.g., Dilantin) that suppress impulse formation
8. Consider use of temporary pacing in case of tachycardias that do not respond to antiarrhythmic drug therapy; these include sustained VT, AV nodal tachycardia, and atrial flutter. In these patients the arrhythmia frequently can be terminated by pacing-induced premature stimuli or pacing above the tachycardia rate.

4. Cation exchange resins (sodium polystyrene sulfonate) by retention enema; this may be repeated until potassium levels are within safe limits. Oral doses of 20 gm are given 3 or 4 times a day together with 20 ml of 70 percent sorbitol solution.
5. If renal failure: hemodialysis or peritoneal dialysis along with one of the treatments above

ECG RECOGNITION OF SEVERE HYPOKALEMIA (SERUM LEVEL OF LESS THAN 2.5 mEq/L)

- ST depression
- Decrease in T wave amplitude
- Increase in U wave amplitude

TREATMENT

1. Potassium chloride IV not to exceed 40 mEq/L at an infusion rate not to exceed 20 mEq/hour (approximately 200 to 250 mEq/day)
2. Oral potassium chloride

insertion; be aware that large hearts and hearts with thick ventricular muscles (as in hypertension) require atrial contribution for adequate systolic output.
2. If pacemaker syndrome is first recognized after implantation, program the rate so that the majority of beats are spontaneous.
3. If unsuccessful, reoperation is necessary for conversion to an atrial pacing device in case of intact atrioventricular (AV) conduction or to a dual chamber unit in case of AV block.

MYOCARDIAL PERFORATION

1. To confirm myocardial perforation, record a unipolar electrogram from the pacing electrode(s); an ECG showing QRS and T waves similar to those recorded on precordial lead V_3 or V_4 indicates that the electrode is outside the heart.
2. Gently withdraw the pacing catheter while recording the ECG from the electrode; in case of a bipolar catheter use the distal electrode! When the QRS complex and T wave are opposite to lead V_3 or V_4, the distal electrode is again inside the right ventricle.
3. In the event of pericardial tamponade, immediate pericardiocentesis and drainage are indicated.
4. Closely monitor the patient.
5. Discontinue anticoagulants.

PACEMAKER-MEDIATED TACHYCARDIA

1. Reprogram the atrial sensing refractory period so that retrograde atrial signals are not sensed.

Emergency Drugs

Table App. 3–1. Intravenous Dosage (Adult) of Drugs Commonly Used During Bradycardia, Tachycardia, or Following Cardiopulmonary Resuscitation*

Drug	Dosage
Adenosine (Adenocard)	6–12 mg
Atropine	0.5–1.0 mg
Bretylium (Bretylol)	2–5 mg/kg
Calcium chloride	500 mg or 6.8 mEq (5 ml of 10% solution)
Digoxin (Lanoxin)	0.125–0.5 mg
Ephedrine	5–10 mg
Epinephrine (Adrenalin)	0.5–1.0 mg
Lidocaine (Xylocaine)	1–1.5 mg/kg bodyweight
Magnesium sulfate or magnesium chloride	1–2 gm (5–10 ml of 20% solution)
Nitroglycerin (Tridil)	200–400 µg
Phenytoin (Dilantin)	100–250 mg IV at 50 mg/min†
Procainamide (Pronestyl)	10 mg/kg/min to 1000 mg
Propranolol (Inderal)	1–2 mg
Sodium bicarbonate	1 mEq/kg
	50–75 ml of 8.4% solution
Verapamil (Isoptin, Calan)	5–10 mg in 2–3 min

*Usually mixed in 5–10 ml D5W or normal saline.
†Use 0.22–0.45 micron filter.

over

Emergency Drugs *Continued*

Table App. 3–3. Dosage of Drugs Used Intravenously for Treatment During Circus Movement Tachycardia Using an Accessory Pathway

Adenosine 6 mg; if unsuccessful 12 mg and may repeat
Verapamil 10 mg over 3 min
Ajmaline 1 mg/kg over 3 min
Procainamide 10 mg/kg over 5 min
Diltiazem hydrochloride 0.25 mg/kg

Table App. 3–4. Dosage of Drugs Used Intravenously for Treatment During Atrial Fibrillation in Patients Using an Accessory Pathway

Procainamide 10 mg/kg over 5 min
Ajmaline 1 mg/kg over 3 min
Disopyramide 1.5 to 2 mg/kg over 5 min

Emergency Axis Determination

RAPID AXIS DETERMINATION

I	II	aVF	
			Normal
			Normal
			Normal
			-30°
			LAD > -30°
			RAD > +120°
			Northwest "No Man's Land"

CHOICE OF ENERGY SETTING

Ventricular Tachycardia. Ten joules (10 J) is usually adequate; 100 J is almost always effective.

Atrial Flutter. Begin with 20 J; energy levels that are too low (5–10 J) may convert atrial flutter to atrial fibrillation. If 20 J is not effective, use 50 or 100 J on repeat attempt.

Supraventricular Tachycardia. Ten joules (10 J) is frequently effective, whereas 100 J is almost always successful.

Atrial Fibrillation. Initial suggested shock strength is 100 J. If not successful, a higher energy shock (200 or 300 J) may be delivered.

Ventricular Fibrillation. Initially 200 J; if unsuccessful this is followed immediately by 350 J. (For children weighing 2.5–50 kg, use 2 J/kg.)

Digitalis Toxicity. In cases of possible or suspected digitalis excess or subclinical digitalis toxicity, it may be safer to start all electrical cardioversion at 5 to 10 J. This may be enough to restore normal sinus rhythm, except in atrial fibrillation, in which case this "test dose" may disclose warning ventricular arrhythmias secondary to subclinical digitalis excess. In this situation the procedure is best terminated and alternative antiarrhythmic therapy planned.

Table App. 3–2. Infusion Mixtures for Drugs Used During Bradycardia, Tachycardia, or Following Cardiopulmonary Resuscitation

Drug	Dose Concentration Per 250 ml D5W	Usual Dose	
		Per ml	Per minute*
Bretylium (Bretylol)	1000 mg	4 mg	1–2 mg
Dobutamine (Dobutrex)	500 mg	2 mg	5–15 μg/kg
Dopamine (Inotropin)	200 mg	800 μg	2.5–20 μg/kg†
Epinephrine (Adrenalin)	1 mg	4 μg	1–8 μg
Isoproterenol (Isuprel)	2 mg	8 μg	1–8 μg
Lidocaine (Xylocaine)	1000 mg	4 mg	1–4 mg
Magnesium sulfate	4 gm	16 mg	16 mg
Nitroglycerin (Tridil, Nitrostat, Nitro-Bid, Nitrocine, Nitrol)	50 mg	200 μg	25–1000 μg
Nitroprusside (Nipride, Nitropress)	50 mg	200 μg	10–500 μg
Norepinephrine (Levophed)	4 mg	16 μg	1–8 μg
Phenytoin (Dilantin)	500 mg	2 mg	200–300 μg
Procainamide (Pronestyl)	1000 mg	4 mg	1–4 mg

*Usually started at a low dose and titrated to desired action. If high doses are used, use higher concentration (×2, ×4) to limit volume of infusion.

†Low dose: 2.5 to 5 μg/kg/min. High dose: (predominant alpha action) 5 to 20 μg/kg/min. For high dose infusion, use a more concentrated solution.

continued